Taekwondo

Your Ultimate Training and Grading Guide

(A Practical Guide to the World's Most Popular Martial Art)

James Johnson

Published By **Zoe Lawson**

James Johnson

All Rights Reserved

Taekwondo: Your Ultimate Training and Grading Guide (A Practical Guide to the World's Most Popular Martial Art)

ISBN 978-1-77485-446-4

All rights reserved. No part of this guide may be reproduced in any form without permission in writing from the publisher except in the case of brief quotations embodied in critical articles or reviews.

Legal & Disclaimer

The information contained in this book is not designed to replace or take the place of any form of medicine or professional medical advice. The information in this book has been provided for educational and entertainment purposes only.

The information contained in this book has been compiled from sources deemed reliable, and it is accurate to the best of the Author's knowledge; however, the Author cannot guarantee its accuracy and validity and cannot be held liable for any errors or omissions. Changes are periodically made to this book. You must consult your doctor or get professional medical advice before using any of the suggested remedies, techniques, or information in this book.

Upon using the information contained in this book, you agree to hold harmless the Author from and against any damages, costs, and expenses, including any legal fees potentially resulting from the application of any of the information provided by this guide. This disclaimer applies to any damages or injury caused by the use and application, whether directly or indirectly, of any advice or information presented, whether for breach of contract, tort, negligence, personal injury, criminal intent, or under any other cause of action.

You agree to accept all risks of using the information presented inside this book. You need to consult a professional medical practitioner in order to ensure you are both able and healthy enough to participate in this program.

TABLE OF CONTENTS

Introduction 1

Chapter 1: An Introduction To Taekwondo And Its Tenets .. 3

Chapter 2: The Basic Stances Of Taekwondo 11

Chapter 3: The Hand Hits 18

Chapter 4: The Kicks 33

Chapter 5: Blocks And Defense Combinations 42

Chapter 6: Counterattacks And Defense 55

Chapter 7: Sport Poomsae 71

Chapter 8: Sparring (Kyroogi) 80

Chapter 9: Weapons 110

Chapter 10: Demonstration Techniques 123

Chapter 11: Bruce Lee's Combat Principles..................... 126

Chapter 12: Combat Principles 133

Chapter 13: Jeet Kune Do Combat Ranges 142

Chapter 14: Punches 148

Chapter 15: Basic Jeet Kune Do Kicks.............................. 157

Chapter 16: Different Kinds Of Tae Kwon Do 165

Chapter 17: Tae Kwon Do Equipment............................. 169

Chapter 18: Tae Kwon Do Kicks And Strikes 172

Chapter 19: The Trainings For Tae Kwon Do 175

Chapter 20: Belts Of Tae Kwon Do 179

Chapter 21: Tae Kwon Do Basics 182

Conclusion 184

Introduction

Taekwondo is a well-known sporting art that is a martial arts. Taekwondo is practiced across more than all 190 countries of the world. In Korea children from as young as 5 years old take taekwondo lessons to build their character as well as protect themselves from attacks that are unlawful.

If you're looking for the right book to educate you about this martial art, and also to teach you the fundamental techniques and drills, then you'll come across this book as an excellent resource.

This book contains the fundamentals you need to learn about Taekwondo by understanding its fundamentals and preparing strategies for fighting. This book can be used to aid you in progressing quicker in taekwondo, and to understand the rules.

This book offers step by procedure execution of drills and strategies that beginners must master. Alongside the procedures, the book includes images to help you understand more clearly and be aware of what can expect from the exercise being covered.

Thank you again for choosing this book . I hope that you will gain a lot of knowledge as we progress.

Chapter 1: An Introduction To Taekwondo And Its Tenets

A Brief Background of Taekwondo

Taekwondo is an Korean martial art believed to be a blend from Taekkyun and Suback two ancient martial arts practices in Korea. Taekwondo literally refers to the way of life with kicks and fists. "Taek" refers to "feet or kick". "Won" is "fist or hand" and "do" is "the lifestyle."

Taekwondo was intended to be a weapon for the ancient Korean soldiers. It was a method to protect themselves in a battle and to win against their adversaries.

In 1945, Taekwondo schools were established in 1945. The first schools didn't take on the name Taekwondo. They were branded with different names as well as taught martial arts in a different way each other. It was not until General Choi Hong-Hi, his students and his colleagues presented their work to Korean president Syngman Rhee in the year 2000 that Taekwondo became acknowledged in the eyes of authorities of the Korean government. President Rhee directed for the martial arts to should be taught to all Korean soldiers in the Korean War.

In recognition of this Taekwondo schools got an upswing. It was in 1955 that the heads of the respective schools, referred to as kwans, decided to join their methods and training to make them more beneficial between them. They initially were referred to as the martial art Tae Soo Do. But General Choi Hong-Hi recommended it that martial arts be named as Taekwondo to put the most importance to one of its mother forms that is the Taekkyun.

In 1973 In 1973, it was in the year 1973 that the World Taekwondo Federation was established. It became the governing body to set the guidelines for the practice of taekwondo as well as the promotion of ranks. They also encourage and regulate studying the art of fighting in more than more than 190 countries around the globe.

Taekwondo as a Sport

Twenty twenty years later, after this martial art was created the art was recognized as an official sport. In 1975, following that the World Taekwondo Federation was established numerous associations and sports clubs recognized Taekwondo as a form of sport.

The 1988 and the 1992 Olympics the sport was only presented for demonstration purposes. The sport was never an official sport. However, because of the growing popularity of the sport and the growing popularity of Taekwondo, the Olympic committee chose to make Taekwondo a formal event. The majority of the athletes who were the most dominant in the sport were Koreans.

Tenets of Taekwondo

The fundamentals of taekwondo are believed to have been originated from the Hwarangdo of the Shilla Dynasty. The hwarangs were soldiers of the elite of Shilla. They were required to go through special training as well as perform important duties. They also had to follow certain important rules. A few of these principles were adopted by Taekwondo.

Taekwondo divided these principles into five fundamental principles. They are:

1. Courtesy (Yom Chi. Taekwondo is a way to teach respect, humility and kindness. Students are required to show respect to their

instructors, to show humility the other students and show kindness to everyone.

Students are required to welcome their teachers, their fellow students as well as the gym or dojo with a bow prior to entering. Also, they must say goodbye to everyone with a bow prior to going out of the dojo.

2. Perseverance (In Nae). Taekwondo is a method of teaching students how to overcome obstacles. They are encouraged to keep training and performing what they are taught despite perceived difficulty, as it is an expression of character and devotion. Therefore, anyone who decides to study martial arts is expected to practice it until the conclusion.

3. Indomitable Spirit (Baekjul Bool Gool). Also, simply speaking, having courage and honor. Taekwondo instructors must give up the most important aspect of their lives, and even their own life, in order to defend the beliefs they hold and what they believe is best overall.

4. Integrity (Yom Chi). Taekwondo constantly reminds the students of being honest both with themselves and with their fellow students. It is not a good idea to cheat during your training or during the fight.

5. Self-control (Guk Gi). Taekwondo realizes that those who are trained in martial arts will frequently be over confident. This is why it teaches its students to be in control regardless of the situation they find themselves in.

It gives two types of self-control. The first one is physical control. This means following the correct method of doing the job, not doing something you're not capable of .

Physical self-control is based on the psychological self-control that is the other type. Taekwondo trains its students to control their emotions, joy, loneliness, and anger. The emotions can influence the way one thinks.

This last rule will allow for an easy implementation of the other four fundamentals. In taekwondo, should you lose control of your own self it is inevitable to lose.

The Taekwondo Commandments

Modern taekwondo has created guidelines that can help students adhere to the principles it seeks to impart. The rules are as the following:

a. Your loyalty to your country

b. Be respectful of your parents

C. Your commitment towards your spouse

D. Remain loyal to your family and friends

It is important to respect your family and friends. Respect your sisters and brothers

f. Respect your elders

G. Respect your teacher

H. Don't take life lightly.

I. Indomitable spirit

j. Your loyalty to your school

K. Do what you began.

Taekwondo versus Karate

At the time that Taekwondo was first introduced there were questions regarding its resemblance to Japan's Karate which also employs kicks and fists for weapons. But, once it was made an actual sport, the differences in the martial art been made clear.

Taekwondo which utilizes four limbs in the fight, was viewed as a two-limb martial art. The use of hands or punches during the game isn't allowed, however it will not earn any points. The kicks alone can earn you points.

Taekwondo Rating and promotion

As with Karate as well as Judo, Taekwondo also uses belts to display the status of the student. Also, it requires a test system to allow the instructor to be promoted. The test could need Kyukpa as well as Poomse.

Kyukpa refers to the technique of breaking. It is taught by adults and older students. It is done by breaking planks or bricks using the feet and hands. Students might have break a specific amount of planks in order to get through the test.

Poomse is the pattern that has been compiled techniques that are used in taekwondo. It is similar to Karate's "Kata" in Karate. The student has to perform several poomse correctly to be able to pass the test.

The student might have be able to pass both tests before they can be promoted. If you are a higher belt the test could require sparring.

The ranking of Taekwondo's belts differs from one school to the next. Certain schools do not have certain colors, however the most basic belts include:

1. White is a color worn by people who aren't so confident.

2. Yellow

3. Orange

4. Green

5. Blue

6. Purple

7. Red

8. Brown

9. Black

The top level in Taekwondo is called the Kwan. The Kwan rank gives you the ability to set up the school in your own.

Chapter 2: The Basic Stances Of Taekwondo

In Taekwondo, and in certain martial arts, stances play a role. Your body posture in general will determine the strength of your feet and hands. If you are in a bad or unbalanced stance and posture, you might not be able to execute the strike correctly and efficiently.

Taekwondo consists of seven stances however only four are suitable for use in an actual self-defense. The rest are employed in competitions, schools as well as when doing the pomse

Non-Fighting Stances

They are used to express respect, and to signal the beginning and the conclusion of the poomse. These stances are moa, charyot, and narani.

Charyot Sogi , or attention Stance

This is the stance that is used when bowing towards the teacher or the dojo. It differs between schools however, these are the steps to follow for that of the Charyot Sogi.

1. Place your feet together and keep your legs straight. The heels should meet and the big toes must be facing each other.

2. Make sure your fist is tightly pressed to your side.

In certain schools, feet aren't placed next to each other. The heel is allowed to be in contact, but the feet are spread out approximately 45 degrees.

Moa Sogi Or Close Stance

The stance is like the charyot or prepared stance, however, it's usually performed after an event. It can also be bowing position. To bow, follow the steps of Charyot Sogi.

Narani Sogi and Ready Stance

The Narani Sogi could be the second posture you take when performing poomse, or simply listening to class. When you are in this position you're in a position to take the order by your instructor. To achieve this position follow these steps.

1. From the charyeot posture then take a step to the side and extend your legs.

2. Straighten your legs. Your fist should be slightly in the direction of your face. Your fist should rest on your shoulders, and they should not touch.

The Fighting Stances

There are four main fighting postures. They are the front stance and the back stance. They are the horse stance, and the rear stance.

The Front Stance or Gunnun Sogi

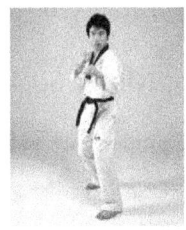

This is an best position to use during competitions or score-based fight. In this position it is possible to have the weight evenly distributed across the legs allowing students the chance to kick with any leg.

For this The steps to take are as follows:

1. From the stance that is ready from the stance, move your dominant foot towards the opposite foot.

2. When you bring your feet towards each the other, you can raise your hand toward your face. Make sure your dominant hand is in a fist, however you can open the other hand.

3. Make sure your dominant leg is farther than the other leg. The legs must be an inch apart.

4. All of your toes should point towards the forward direction. Your shoulder should be straight to ensure stability of your legs.

The Back Stance or Niunja Sogi

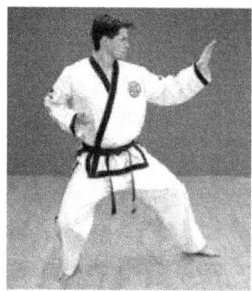

The back stance is an excellent posture to prepare to help you kick your rear legs with power or hand strikes. It lets your hips expand, bringing the power of your legs.

These are steps to take for this position:

1. Follow the steps 1 and 2 of the front stance.

2. Move your dominant leg to the southeast position, if you are right-handed. If you're left-handed then pull your leg towards your southwest position. Your distance must be around an inch apart.

3. Your toes should face towards the side, while the opposite foot stays pointed towards the front. Your legs should be in an L-shaped shape.

4. Your hips should be pulled towards the dominant leg. The weight should be placed on your back foot. Bend your knees to gain greater balance and force.

The Rear Foot Stance, or Bom Sogi (Tiger Stance)

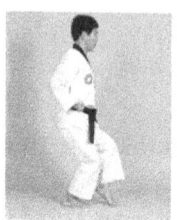

The stance of the rear foot is the result of the back stance and front stance. Contrary to the front stance the weight isn't equally distributed between the legs. In the rear foot stance, most of the weight falls located on the rear leg that's the same as that of the back posture. But, unlike the back stance, the foot of the rear is placed in front of that of the foot in front. It is shorter.

Here are some ways to comprehend more clearly:

1. Follow all the steps in the front posture.

2. Bring your hips up to your rear as if you're planning to sit.

3. Move your front leg towards your back foot. Bend your knees. Keep your back foot flat on the floor . Keep your front foot elevated with the soles of your feet resting on the ground.

Horse Stance or Annun Sogi

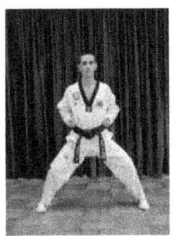

The horse's stance is rarely employed in a taekwondo contest because it is best suited for punches. It is the most basic posture that is used in Kyukpa because it allows for a smooth transfer of power to the top area of the body. These are the steps to follow:

1. Make sure you are in the position to be ready.

2. Bring your dominant leg toward the other leg. You may take this step off in case you prefer. However, it is recommended to keep your posture in check.

3. Do not lift your hands in front of your face. Instead, put them into the shape of a fist, and then place them next to your fist.

4. Transfer your legs to the side about 1 and half of your shoulder length. Bend your knees and pull your butt in the same way as if you're straddling the back of a horse.

Chapter 3: The Hand Hits

Taekwondo is a sport that has two types of hand strike. Each strike is dependent on the hand's position. The first is an open hand strike, and the other type is close hand strike.

Taekwondo is an athletic discipline hand strikes are not able to bring any points in the course of the fight. They earn points only when a poomse or kyukpa contest is held and the demonstrations.

However, in self-defense strategy, the hand strikes can be used as a knife or weapon for an individual. Here are a few most basic hand strikes, depending on the hand's position.

Strikes with open hands

Sahnkal and Knifehand Strike

Picture sourced from www.wikipedia.com

The knifehand strike uses your hand as an asymmetrical sword. The typical knifehand strike employs the edge of your hand, specifically the area just below the little finger and over the wrist to hit the opponent. If it is done correctly and hits precisely it could cause the opponent to fall asleep. The most common target for the knife is the throat.

For preparing your hand to be your knifehand you just need to follow two steps.

1. Put your thumb in the middle the thumb and then

2. Make sure your fingers are tightly to one another. Your pressure must be at the outside of your hand.

There are two types that knifehands strike. They are the outside knifehand as well as the knifehand inside. To show the difference following steps for each strike:

The Outside Knifehand

1. In the back stance position.

2. Both hands should be in the knifehands position.

3. Your rear hand should be pulled to the back from your neck. Your palm should be pointing towards your opponent . Your shoulders should pull toward the back. Lift your left hand higher than your head. It is possible the hand raised higher in case your opponent is larger than you are.

4. Your hand should be lowered while you snap your wrist towards the inside. You can twist your hips while you swing to get more strength. Also, you must move your front foot toward the outside.

This is the Inside Knifehand Strike

1. Make sure you are in the combat stance and extend your hands to your knifehand position.

2. Your hand should be pulled back towards your shoulder in front. Your elbow should line up with your nose. Your thumb should be in the area below your ears.

3. In a chopping swing then pull your hand toward your opponent.

4. Your elbow, fingers as well as shoulder must be in alignment to hit your goal to increase your strength.

If you are in self-defense, attack your adversary on the eye's side (temple). This can cause a decrease in his vision , and could allow you to escape. If you wish to get him to fall, strike him in the throat.

Oppun Sahnkhal as well Ridgehand Strike

Oppun Sahnkhal Oppun Sahnkhal represents the reverse from the position of the knife. Instead of striking you opponent by using area below the finger, you strike him with the portion that runs from your index finger until your wrist.

Similar to knives, the hand comes with the inside as well as the outside strike. The steps are described in the following paragraphs:

A Ridgehand's Outside Position

1. Follow the steps 1 through 3 of the knifehand outside position.

2. Your hands should be pointing towards the target, but do not snap your wrist. Your hips should be twisted as you move your arms. Turn your foot towards the outsidetoo.

3. Your elbow, hand and shoulder ought to be in alignment when you reach your goal.

Aside Ridgehand Pose

1. Follow the steps 1 through 2 of the knifehand's inside position.

2. Your hands should be pointing towards your goal while slapping your wrist towards the inside.

The rigdehand strike may not be as effective than the knifehand strike but hitting the correct target may make your opponent weaker. The ideal option for this strike is the area that lies between your chin and neck.

Sahn Deung Backhand Strike

The sahn dung is similar to reverse slap. Instead of slapping your palm, you'll be slapping using the side part of your hands. The part that strikes your opponent could seem to represent the part that runs from your knuckles to your wrist, however the real portion you should be hitting is the knuckles of your index and middle fingers.

The most common target for the attack is the jaw as well as the cheeks.

For your backhand strike you must follow these steps.

1. Take a frontal stance.

2. Place your back hand in your ear's front. Your palm should be facing your head while your thumb should be level with your ears.

3. Your hand should be swung in an upward direction, but do not alter the hand's position.

4. Stretch your hand to the max. Fingers should remain in line with your elbow and shoulders.

5. You can twist your body and rear foot while swinging to boost your force.

Kwan Soo, or Spearhand Strike

Image taken from wikiwand.com

A spearhand strike called"hand thrust. It follows the knifehand posture however, the three fingers that are taller are the ones that strike the target. This is a perfect hand strike, but it is able to be more effective at hitting pressure points. It is able to strike the windpipe as well as also the solar plexus. All of these points can cause the victim to lose breath or in a state of sleep.

Below are some steps to follow for the spearhand strike.

1. Step into an asymmetrical rearfoot stance, or the back stance.

2. Your dominant hand should be pulled open to the point that it is just above your waistline.

3. Take a step forward using your back foot. Bring your hand forward with the direction of a swinging motion. Make sure to extend your hand completely. You can twist your body while you push to increase the strength. You can strike your palms upwards, downwards or sideways.

Bahtong Sahn or Palm Heel Strike

Bahtong Sahn strikes your opponent with the palm's heel. This hand strike requires you be more close to the opponent. It also requires some momentum from your side.

The most common target for this kind of strike is the cheeks. If you're in the dirt, then you may use this technique to strike the region of the groin. It's also a great technique to push your opponent off.

To perform the proper palm heel strike For correct palm heel strike, follow these steps to follow.

1. Take a rear or the back position.

2. As you place your feet, you should open both hands and reduce your dominant hand to just over your waist.

3. Clap your fingers in your dominant hand half way and then form the bear claw. Your wrist should be bent to the back.

4. Then, you can thrust your hand in a diagonal upward direction. When you are thrusting, turn your wrist towards the inside. Your palm should be facing the opponent.

5. Hit your opponent with the palm's heel.

Close Hand Strikes

Close-hand strikes can be done exactly the same way as open hand strikes, however, your hands are closed to different positions for your fists. Below is a discussion of each of the different fist positions.

Joomuk and the Fist

Photo taken from www.livestrong.com

The joomuk is the correct weapon employed in Taekwondo. For this simply move your fingers towards your palm. Put your thumb below the middle of the knuckles of your middle and index fingers.

The middle knuckles on all of your fingers should be in an uniform line. The top knuckles on your middle and index fingers are higher than those of the other two fingers. The upper knuckles of your fingers and your middle knuckles are slightly less than 90 degrees in alignment.

Deung Joomuk, or Back Fist

In deung joomuks your hands will follow the direction of the joomuk. The only difference is the part that hits the area of the target. When you use the deung joomuk you'll use the upper back of your knuckles specifically the forefinger as well as the middle finger knuckles.

Yup Joomuk, or the side fist

The Yup joomuk follows the same joomuk position but it is played using only the edges of your hand, or the area below the wrist and little finger.

My Joomuk or the Hammer fist

Me Joomuk is a fist that is vertical. Instead of aligning your knuckles to the side, they're directed downwards with your thumb on the bottom. The hammer fist can only be employed by swinging your hands in a vertical direction. The lower part of the fist is aimed at the goal.

Inju Joomuk or Forefinger One-Knuckle fist

Image taken from Wikipedia.com. Wikipedia.com

Inju Joomuk strikes your opponent with your forefinger. To get to this hand position you need to follow these steps.

1. Make sure you hold your hands in one fist.

2. You can roll the index finger out about halfway. Your middle knuckle must be in alignment with the rest of your arms.

Bamju Joomuk, or middle Finger one-knuckle fist

The same principle applies to the inju joomuk. However, instead of rolling your forefinger, instead you extend your middle finger.

After you've learned the fundamental fist position and the techniques for punching used in Taekwondo.

Combinations and Punching Techniques Utilizing the Close Hand Positions

Here are some of the fundamental and most popular techniques for punching in taekwondo.

Bahru Chirugi, or Straight Punch

Bahru Chirugi is aiming his punch towards the middle. It is a straight strike that is, it's directed towards the middle of the torso of the opponent. It is also possible to execute in a downward or upward direction that are known as jae-chuh chirugi or nehryu in their respective terms. It is possible to use any combat posture to perform this punch.

When you throw your punch, your elbow, fist and shoulders are in alignment to each other. Your armpit does not open wide.

The typical target of this type of punch is the face windpipe, solar plexus, face and the groin.

Gullgi Chirugi, or Hook Punch

Gullgi Chirugi is striking towards the center from outside. The most common target of this attack is the face's side jaw, the face and the ribs.

To accomplish this, follow these steps to follow.

1. Take on any fighting stance.

2. Make sure you keep your dominant fist (or the front fist) at a level that is just beyond your waist. The palm's heel should be facing upwards.

3. Bring your elbow up to nearly equalize your shoulder. While you raise it, bend your wrist towards the inside.

4. Take your hands from the outside and place your fist directly on the target.

Chi Chirugi or Uppercut Punch

Image taken from the website. Taekwondo.wikia.com

Uppercuts are similar to the palm-heel stike but instead of striking your opponent by putting your heel into his palm, you strike the person by using your fist. The focus of it is your chin, and it is also known as the solar plexus. It's also one of the momentum punches. It is important to determine the perfect timing for it.

Here are the steps needed to follow.

1. Take any fight stance however, a an inclination to the back is suggested.

2. Once you have reached your stance, slowly move your dominant hand or the one you are holding towards your side, just below your waist. The palm's heel should be facing upwards.

3. Your fist is pushed in an upward direction.

4. Bend your knees , and then arch your back while you kick the punch to get greater power.

Doo Joomuk Chirugi or Double Fist Punch

Doo Joomuk Chirugi can land your punches at the same time in one spot. It's a punch with momentum that requires precision and timing. It is necessary to stand in a horse's stance in order for the correct execution of the punch.

The punch could be straight or hook, or it can be an uppercut.

Dikootja Chirugi or Chirugi or "U" and "C" Punch

Dikootja Chirugi is at the same time throwing straight punches with either an upward or downward punch.

To accomplish this follow these steps, here are the steps:

1. Take a horse's stance and stand in it.

2. Change to front or back stance while you move one hand to your upper center, and the other one to you middle middle.

3. Then, you can push your fists up, striking two targets.

Doo Bun Chirugi or Double Punch

Doo bun chirugi throws two consecutive punches at one area. It is typically used after an attack. Also, you should not alter your posture when you throw the punches. The typical punches that are used to create this double punch include the straight one along with the punch for uppercuts.

Sae Bun Chirugi or Triple Punch

Sae Bun is throwing three straight punches in succession without altering your posture. The straight punch that is upwards is first thrown.

When you are pulling your hands back to your waist, it is time to throw your middle straight strike using the other hand. When you bring it back towards your waist you will throw downward straight punch with your first hand.

Chapter 4: The Kicks

Taekwondo is renowned because of its kicks. In contrast to karate and others martial arts, it employs more kicks as opposed to the hands. Hands are considered to be swords, whereas Taekwondo kicks are regarded as the spears.

In the end, in Taekwondo as a game, only the kicks score. Here are a few fundamental kicks that beginners should be able to master.

Ahp Chagi and Front Kick

Front kicks are similar to the straight punch that you can do with your feet. You move your feet toward the center, straight upwards as well as straight back. The part which hits the goal is the toes' ball. It's the part of your feet that is beneath your big toe and below the second toe.

It is among the kicks targeted at the face, the chin the windpipe, and solar plexus.

Here are step by procedure for a perfect front kick.

1. Engage in any fighting stance however, a back kick is the preferred choice. For kick combinations front stance as well as the rear stance are better.

2. Put your hands slightly ahead of your face. Your hand in front should be in an open position and the other hand must be in a closed hand position.

3. Let's suppose that you're doing a kick with your rear leg. Move your knee to the rear and out to the front. The knee must be 90 degrees to your body. Your feet should be 90 degrees to your shin.

4. Lower your leg and kick it up to strike your desired target. When you kick, move your hips, then turn your front leg towards the outside, aiming for 45 degrees.

Yup Chig, or Side Kick

Yup chagi can be described as placing your foot in the position of a knife. The area that strikes on the goal is actually the top that your feet are, or the part below your little toe to your heel. To perform this kick correctly Here are the steps to follow.

The typical target of this kind of kick is the chin, face, the windpipe as well as the solar plexus.

1. The steps are 1 and 2. Follow them to the kick position.

2. Bring your knee up to your back and turn your front foot outwards towards 90 degrees. When you twist your foot then swing your hips towards the center. Your body will appear to be facing the direction of your front foot.

3. Lengthen your leg towards the side. Widening your thighs for greater power and to maintain your stability.

Dolrya Chagi, or Round House Kick

This is by far the most commonly used kick in Taekwondo or any martial art that utilizes kicks. It is referred to as the most powerful kicks. The area of your foot that hits the target is called the instep, or the portion of your foot that is between your toes and your front ankle.

The main targets in the roundhouse kick are the sides of your head jaw, and the ribs. Below are some steps to accomplish it.

1. Find your stance for fighting. If you are looking for a strong roundhouse, try your back position.

2. Your hands should be slightly in front of your face. Your hand in front should be in an open position and the other must be in a closed hand position.

3. Bring your knee up to bring your hips level. Your knee and your body should be 90 degrees. Your toes must be pointed toward the floor.

4. Turn your front foot towards the outside around 45 degrees.

5. When you move your foot around, turn your rear hip slightly until 45 degrees. Bring your knee back to a degree and pull your rear foot and shin out.

6. You can move your leg from the front, and then twist your hips 90 degrees.

Bahndall Chagi as well as Cresent Kick

Crescent kicks are nearly original and is only available for Taekwondo. In many martial arts it is not possible to receive a score. However, they do in Taekwondo. It's just as important as other kicks.

The crescent kick is nearly similar to the slap kick. However the kick is thrown from outside or the inside, not from the center. The crescent kick comes in two forms. There is an inside crescent kick as well as the external crescent kick. To comprehend the crescent kicks more clearly follow these steps for each kind:

Outside Crescent Kick

1. Find your fighting position. Also, a back stance is the best choice.

2. Put your hands in the typical position described above.

3. Turn your hips and foot by between 45 and 90 degrees, and then swing your leg towards the target at the same time. Your kick should start by keeping your knees in a straight position. Don't curl like your previous ones. Your foot should be drawing the final quarter moon.

4. To kick the outside of your crescent make use of either the balls of your foot or your heel to strike the target.

Inside Crescent kick

1. Make sure you are in a fighting stance. To perform this crescent kick the rear foot stance is the best choice.

2. Put your hands in the typical position previously discussed.

3. While not twisting your front foot or your hips, kick your knees straight and in an upward

diagonal move similar to drawing the first quarter moon. If your goal is high, then you can put your front foot into the tiptoe position.

4. Your hips should be turned to the opposite side and let your foot drop onto your goal. To get the best results, hit your target using the edge that your feet are, which is the portion below your smallest toe and the heel.

Chigo Chagi or Axe Kick

The axe kick is a unique kick, yet it is the best kick in taekwondo combat. It's unusual in that the strike does not come from the middle or on the side, but instead from the top. Axe kicks can leave your opponent exhausted or even knocked out completely If you execute the kick properly.

Below are some steps to follow to create an axe kick that is powerful.

1. Make sure you are in a fighting stance. The ideal stance for this kick is to take the front position.

2. While keeping the knee bent, you can lift your back leg over the head of your opponent. You may slouch when you raise your leg. Your

front foot could be on tiptoes to allow for a more powerful kick.

3. Your foot should fall on the head of your opponent, causing it to hit him. When you are pulling your foot downwards, your aim is to smash your opponent. Retract your lower body while you lower your leg to increase your power.

Dwi Chagi as well as Back Kick

Kicking back is yet another kick that demands the use of momentum and precision. It is important to execute it properly and at the right moment to cause maximum harm to the opponent. This isn't a dangerous strike, however it could send your opponent flying across the space.

These are steps to the best back kick.

1. Make sure you are in a fighting posture. A back foot stance as well as a rear posture are great for this.

2. Turn your front foot 180 degrees. Allow your hips to follow the twist of your foot.

3. As you turn your hips then bend your knee towards your stomach. Your toes should be pointed towards the floor.

4. Straighten your knee so that it hits the goal with your back. Then, bend your head and go lower it a bit to raise the kick.

Miro Chagi or Push Kick

Push kicks are not an attack kick. It's a defensive or offensive method. If the opponent you're facing is trying get you cornered and push you, you can do it by using this kick. It's similar with the kick that you use in front. The only difference is the location of the foot and knee as well as the intent to harm your opponent.

To do the correct push kick For a proper push kick, follow these steps to follow.

1. Find your fighting posture. However, you don't necessarily require a correct position to kick a push.

2. Then lift your knee towards your chest, then move your lower leg so that you can place your foot against the stomach or chest of your opponent.

3. Straighten your knee quickly and push away your opponent.

Gawhi Chagi or Scissor Kick

Gawgu Chagi, also known as a double kick that is used to kick opponents in opposite directions simultaneously. It's also known by the name double kick.

In order to do this properly You must be able to climb to the highest point you are able. The steps needed to perform these jumps can be found here.

1. Take a stance that is ready.

2. Reduce your hips and bent your knees. Do as high as you are able to.

3. While you jump, toss your legs around in different directions. Your feet's position can be side kicks as well as a mix of forward and a back kick.

Chapter 5: Blocks And Defense Combinations

Taekwondo is a self-defense martial art. Therefore, it focuses on blocking strikes from your opponent. But, blocking isn't the only thing vital. It is equally important that you are able to defend yourself against attacks to allow you more chances to get away or escape your attacker. This chapter we'll be discussing the various blocking techniques and integrate these techniques into defense combos to help defend yourself.

The most fundamental rule of blocking methods is to place the force in your forearm, not your hand or fist. Your forearm acts as your shield.

Makhikhi or Blocking Poses Makhi

Ahnuro Maki, or Inside Block

Ahnuro Maki blocks the strike of your opponent with your forearm's outer part. It's a great block against punches and other attacks that are directed towards the middle in your. To effectively block with the inward block take these steps.

Let's assume that your opponent throws an unidirectional punch at your chest.

1. Retire in a back stance posture.

2. Bring your front hand up to your face at an angle of 45 degrees. Your rear hand should be under your ear as if you were about to kick your face.

3. Take your wrist and snap it in and move your forearm around your body or face. Make sure you push your opponent's inner forearm towards you. When you shift your back forearm the table, move your forearms forward toward your earlobe in the rear. The hand position will appear like an unbalanced "x". This is the ideal position for a block that is outward when your opponent hits you with a follow-up strike.

4. Lean back a bit while you try to block your opponent in order to stay away from him.

Bakhuro Maki, or Outward Block

Bakhuro Maki blocks the strike by using your forearms, primarily using your wrist. This is a great method of preventing hook and roundhouse kicks that strike the face. Below are some steps to follow.

Let's say that your opponent throws a cross-punch from his rear hand.

1. In a back stance, retreat. posture.

2. Put your forearms in front of you towards your face at about 45 degrees. Maintain your back arm close to your waist.

3. Then, turn your wrist to the side and move your forearm toward the outside. Reflect the forearm from your foe by pushing his internal forearm back away from the body..

4. When you are pushing the strike of your opponent away, turn your hips, and then push your body towards your dominant side just a bit. This is so that you can maintain your distance to the hand you are holding. The strike of your opponent could be powerful enough to cause you to pull back your forearm. Should your head be nearer than your forearm and you are able to strike your face with your block.

Cho Kyo Maki, Rising/Upward block

Upward blocks block the vertical strikes of your opponent, like the axe strike. They also help to deflect strikes toward your face. For you to execute this block in the correct design, follow these steps.

1. In a back stance, retreat. posture.

2. Your forearm should be placed at 45 degrees in front of your face.

3. Relax your knees behind slightly and then turn your wrist to the outside and then raise your forearm slightly and away off your face. When you are pushing your forearm forward and down, you can pull the opposite arm toward your waist.

4. The back of your head should be slightly rounded to stay away from the blocking hand. You don't want your hand to bounce off and strike your forehead.

This is the proper way that is used for upward blocks. However, many instructors recommend moving the front of your foot inwards, and blocking your opponent's forearms with your upper, instead of using your back to arch. This will stop him from making a new attack at you.

You can also reverse your back rather than making your spine arch. This will allow you to have the proper distance to kick. But, it also gives your opponent the chance to launch an additional strike.

Ahrae Maki or block Low/Downward

Downward blocks can be a powerful method of avoiding the strikes or kicks of your opponent towards you lower body. It's like an inward blocks, however the forearm extends lower. These are steps you need to follow to effectively utilize this downward block.

1. Return to the back stance.

2. Let your knees bend a bit.

3. Place your hand on your face at an angle of 45 degrees.

4. Your rear fist should be placed just below your ear. Keep your wrist in the outside and then the entire rear forearm downwards. Your forearm should be aligned with your knee in front.

5. When you pull your back hand, extend your front arm towards your hips.

6. When you are attempting to push your opponent away, you should move your body back to stay away from the attack even if your hand isn't able to stop it.

It is also the most appropriate shape that the block is in the direction of downwards. But, you can also learn the sliding techniques learned in the upper block.

Gahwi Makhi, or Scissor Block

Gawhi Makhi is a combination of the down block and the outside block. The two blocks are performed in tandem. This is referred to as a scissor block since your hands intersect one another like the scissor when you perform the block. For a better understanding of the block, these steps are:

1. Reverse into your position.

2. Put your hands in front of you at 45 degrees. It should be slightly behind your face. Your rear hand should be placed upon your hips. Bend your knees.

3. Your front wrist should be snagged into the opposite direction and perform the outside block using your hands in front. When you turn your wrist in front, you can also twist your rear wrist to the side and pull your rear hand downwards in an outside downward direction.

Your hands in the front is supposed to be aligned in line with the front knee and your hand on the back should be sit in line with your back knee.

4. Turn your body to the dominant side, and push the body back away from the hand in front while you block. This will increase the strength of your blocks.

Yeot Pero Makhi, or "X" Block

"X" block "X" block comes with two variants. There is both the lower "x" block as well as ascending "x" block. This block is ideal to stop vertical kicks either downward or upward vertical kicks. Here is the fundamental form of an "x" block for each type of kick.

Lower "X" Block

1. In a back stance, retreat. posture.

2. Expand both arms to make an x "x".

3. lower your "x" by bent knees. Your hips should be twisted a bit to move your body toward the forward. Your back foot could be tipped-toed. Make sure your knees are bent.

4. Make sure to place your front foot just a bit in front of the block. The reason for this is to be able to easily perform knee blocks if your opponent's kick passes through the block, and/or to quickly respond by kicking forward

after you have deflected the kick of your opponent.

Moving up or down "X" Block

1. Follow the steps 1. and 2. above.

2. Lower your knees and bend them lower. Your back will arch as you lift an "x" Block slightly over your head.

3. Your fist should be aligned to your knees in front. This will ensure that the palm of your hands is securely kept away from your head.

Daebi Makhi, or Guarding Block as well as Double Block

Daebi Makhi is a second two-hand block made of two hands. It is usually performed with fingers in the knifehand, but it could also be performed in the fist position. This is a great option if you are less powerful than your opponent, and blocking with just one hand might not suffice. It's also a good option for those who prefer punch more often than punch.

These are steps needed to build the most effective block to guard against.

1. Make sure you are in your back in a back stance.

2. Put your hands on your shoulder in front. It is possible to use the knifehand position or hand position with your fingers in the fist. Your hand in front should be less than 90 degrees to your shoulder. Your hand behind should be a little under your chin or directly over your chest.

Your front hand should be facing to the side, while you palms of your back hand should be facing up.

3. The wrist of your hand on the inside. Twist the wrists of your back hand towards the outside. Bring both hands toward your ear.

4. Move forward with your back leg, then drop your hands down in a diagonal direction or in a cutting motion.

Sahntol Makhi or the Mountain Block.

The Mountain block can be described as an outside block using both of your forearms. It's actually utilized to open close double hands attack, e.g. doublefist punches. It is also a good option for when two opposing players are striking or directly at you. Below are some steps.

1. Retire from a horse's stance.

2. Your fists should be over your waist.

3. Your wrists should be turned to the inside, and then cross your forearms towards the middle the body. Your hands should rest below your nose.

4. Your hands should be pulled to the outside and away from one another. Your elbows should be aligned with your knees, and your palms should face upwards.

5. Your shoulder blades should be closer to one another to boost your strength.

Palm Block or Hook Block Technique

The palm block is similar to the other four blocks however, rather than a fist the hand is placed in an unlocked palm. It is not used to block an opponent, however, it is used to secure the hand of your opponent. In a sense the palm block isn't actually a block. It's a type of parrying.

Here's how it's done.

For the palm block on the outside:

1. In a back-to-back stance, stand.

2. Make sure your fist is in a 45 degrees to your face.

3. If your opponent is striking then twist your wrist to the side. While you twist, you can extend your palm into the "c" place.

4. Grab your opponent's forearm, keep it in place and pull it forward in a downward direction.

For the palm block on the inside:

1. Follow the initial three steps of the palm block on the outside.

2. Take the forearm of your opponent and keep it in place and move it in an upward direction.

To use the downward and upward block, follow the instructions to make the palm block inside however, you must push your opponent's hand towards the downward and upward direction, respectively.

Scooping Block

Scooping block is a different parrying block. It's sometimes referred to as crescent blocking. It is based on the same blocking techniques, however you move your hands around like you're steering the wheel. The goal is that you throw the opponent's hands away from you, instead of stopping his attack.

Blocks can provide you with the momentum needed to perform momentum-based attacks like back kicks or back fists. It also gives you a the chance to get the circular kick, crescent kick as well as a side kick.

It is possible to do this with the outside and the inside of the block. These are the steps to follow:

To make to use the Outward Block for Scooping:

1. Take a back stance, or any other vertical fighting stance.

2. Slide your hand from the rear onto your opposite side and turn the hand outwards with as much force as you are able to. The goal is typically the upper forearm.

3. While you are steering your hand, turn your shoulder in the same manner to increase your force.

To make the inward scooping block:

1. Make sure you are in your back stance, or any other stance for fighting that is vertical.

2. Move your hands from outside towards the inside. It's similar that the block on your inside however your forearm faces away towards your body. The focus is still on the upper forearm.

3. While you control your hand, make an incline with your back foot. Additionally, you can use similarly to give additional power.

Chapter 6: Counterattacks And Defense

Once you have mastered the fundamental block and attack, here are some basic defense and counterattack strategies that you can utilize to give yourself the opportunity to knock down your opponent , or even escape.

How to Protect Yourself from Axes and Kicks

Single hand block and Knifehand Combination

The single handblocks and knifehand combo is among the most fundamental, yet effective self-defense techniques in Taekwondo. Here's how it's performed.

Block outside Outside block Knifehand Combination

Step 1: Remain to your back stance or in any stance of fighting.

Step 2 Step 2: Block your opponent's attack by using the outside of your block. While you block, raise your fist in an open-handed position and then strike your opponent's neck, on the opposite side of the side that is striking.

This action could cause your opponent to fall. If he isn't able to slide or weaken then you can add these additional actions.

Step 3: Unlock your hand to block and twist into a scooping posture. You can twist your wrist towards the outside and then hold the hand of your opponent.

Fourth step: Quickly draw your hand toward you. When you are pulling closer, you can pull him back with your hand to the rear as you throw an inward knifehand hit to the opposite side of his neck.

If this does not cause him to retreat to the side, try adding the basic throw of taekwondo.

To perform the throw in taekwondo, these are how to do it.

Basic Throwdown and Sweep Taekwondo

Step 1: Keep grabbing the hand of your opponent. Bring him closer. Put a hand on his back on the other shoulder.

Step 2 Step 2: Move your body towards your opponent. Then, you can pull your opponent toward his back, causing him to lose his balance.

Step 3. Slide your back foot towards the back of his knee in front. Kick or swivel the rear of his front knee while you push him downwards.

Step 4: Once you are on the ground, hand him a straight downward punch to his throat, face or chest.

To help you understand the steps for understanding the steps, here's an illustration to help you understand the steps.

Inside block Inside block Knifehand Combination

The steps for this combination are similar to the previous combo, but the hand positions for the opponent are different. These are the steps to follow:

Step 1. Stand in one of the fighting stances however, back and rear postures are the most preferable.

Step 2. Block your opponent's front hand.

Step 3: Spread your back hand and place it over your head. Drop the knifehand on his neck. same side where he has struck his hand.

Step 4: If he is not weaken, grasp your hand close and pull him back. When you pull him close take a scoop of your back hand and place it over your head, and then offer him another smack to the opposite side of his neck.

The 5th step: If you'd like to go even further, you can add a throw to the end.

Block as well as Double Punch combination

A second defense option is to double punch and block combination. It doesn't require any the use of a holding technique, and it may not be able to knock your opponent out however, it could allow you to establish the right distance to strike. It is also a good tool to aid you in escaping.

This combo can be made with the outside, inside blocks, upward and downward. These are the steps to follow:

Step 1 Step 1: Stand in the stance of the back. In addition, any stance of fighting is a good choice.

Step 2 Make sure you block your attacker's strikes by using the correct block as described above.

Step 3. Take the forearm of your opponent (optional). Make a slight step back from the hand of your opponent. Take his hand off and punch him twice on his stomach, ribs or chest.

Based on this you can finish it off with a simple roundhouse kick with your front foot.

Variation: Instead , of the double punch, you could make use of Triple punch. But, it is important to be quick when you execute the punches, as your opponent could take advantage of an opportunity to strike attack at you.

You could also include a front kick or roundhouse kick towards near the top of your set.

Palm Block Kick, Palm Block, and Straight Punch

This is a basic strategy that you should master. It may not cause the most damage to your opponent, however, it's a great strategy to to get away from your adversaries. These some steps.

Use the palm block with the outside:

Step 1: Take your stance of fighting.

Step 2: Counter your opponent's strike by using the outside palm block. Take hold of his forearm.

Step 3. Step 3: Walk sideways towards the front using your rear foot . Throw a roundhouse kick onto the stomach or on higher. Then follow it up by punching straight into the ribs or in the face.

Utilizing the palm block on the inside:

Step 1: Take your stance on your back.

Step 2: Block your opponent's punch by using the inside block, and then grab his forearm.

Step 3. Pull your opponent in close, and then hit him with an uppercut on the solar plexus , or his chin.

Sidestep Sparring Technique

A way to defend yourself is by avoiding the strikes of your opponent, particularly the kicks. The most effective way to avoid striking is to slip towards your adversary. This technique is known as the sidestep. It is a great method to put your opponent hurt while you attempt to get away.

Here are a few most basic sidestep strategies:

Sidestep Roundhouse Kick

This is a good technique to apply when your opponent is kicks using their back foot. Here's how to accomplish it.

1. Take the stance the opponent. This will allow you to figure out the direction he'd attach to your stance and how you should move. Make sure you make a sidestep in where the ball is going, and not in opposition to it.

2. If your opponent is throwing an elbow with his back foot, move into an upward diagonal direction using your front foot.

3. The result will be an stance in which your front foot is now the rear one. Utilizing your stance with this foot you can throw the roundhouse kick onto the back of your opponent.

Turn Sidestep, and Roundhouse kick

Flip sidestep is one of the variants of side step. In this case, you take one side step, then switch your body towards the other side. It is possible to flip it 90 or 180 degrees. The difference between both the sidestep flip and regular sidestep is that the stance is not altered.

This is a good way to stay clear of frontal kicks. The steps are explained in the following paragraphs:

1. Make sure you are in a fighting stance.

2. If your opponent is throwing either a front kick or an Axe kick, make one step back with you frontfoot.

3. Turn your front foot the inside , then throw your back foot towards the rear to your forward foot. You'll still maintain your original posture, however your position will be flipped 90-180 degrees from the original place.

4. Utilizing your rear foot to make a kick in the roundhouse towards the stomach or to his face. If you are able to do triple kicks or double kicks, then you can do the same.

The Basics Two Step Blocking Technique and Counter Attack

When they step, it is two strikes performed by two separate steps. Step sparring is generally used to do point sparring. But, it could be an effective defense. There are two steps to counter-attacks and blocking you could employ.

Outside Block, Cross Block, Double Fist Combination

This combo is a great defensive option for straight punches as well as frontal kick.

The situation and steps to take are the following:

1. He is in a combat posture. You can copy his posture.

2. He will step forward using his rear foot, and then throw straight at you. If you see him, move back, you should retreat to your front stance, and take the strike with an outside block.

3. Your opponent will respond to your unsuccessful strike by kicking him in the front. Your front foot in front of your rear foot, then do an opposite front stance using your legs. When you are ready to return for the stance, you should do your down "x" block.

4. Put your fists in a row and then throw two fists to your foe. Below is an illustration of the combo.

Double Block, Outward Palm Block and Roundhouse Kick Combination

In this scenario your opponent will throw the ball, as well as punch. Here is the scenario as well as the steps to follow for application of the technique.

1.   Your opponent throws a roundhouse kick using his rear foot. You take a side step with your front foot if you are standing in the vertical stance, e.g., front stance. If you are standing in horse stance, just move your foot, opposite of the kicking leg, backward and assume a front or rear stance.

2.   Block the kick using a double block with both your outer foreams.

3.   Your opponent will follow his failed kick with a hook punch using his front hand. Slide your front foot to the back and reverse your original stance.

4.   As you reverse your stance, block the punch using the outward palm block. Hold his hand and pull him close.

5.   As you pull him close, throw a roundhouse kick to his stomach, face or chest.

Below is a step by step illustration of the combination.

Basic Three Step Sparring

Three blocks and a Punch Combination

In this situation, your opponent is attacking you with three punches. You are to defend with three outside blocks and counter attacking with a straight punch. To explain further, here are the steps:

1. Your opponent will throw straight or hook punches at you. He will take a step forward as he throws a punch.

Block his punches with outside blocks. Retreat to alternate front stance every time you block your opponent and block with alternate hands.

2. On the last outside block, shift to back stance and throw a straight punch at your opponent.

To understand better, here is an illustration for you.

Variation: Instead of outside block, you can do inside blocks.

Instead of a single punch, you can extend it to double punch or three way punches. You may also do the front kick with your rear foot instead of the punch.

Three downward blocks and a Front kick Combination

For this combination, we will assume that your opponent is attacking you with three front kicks. You will defend yourself by blocking his kicks with downward blocks and counter with a front kick, too.

Here are the scenarios and the steps you should do:

1.   Your opponent will strike you with a front kick. You will block it with a downward block. Every time you block it, he will drop his kick outside or between your legs to close the distance between you.

Thus, every time you block the kick, take a step back and retreat to a front stance.

2.   On your last block, shift to rear or back stance and throw a front kick with your front foot.

To understand the steps better, see the illustrations below.

Variations:

Instead of your front foot, use your rear foot. You can also throw a roundhouse kick with your rear foot.

Instead of a kick, you can throw double or triple punch combination. You can also counter with a knifehand strike on his neck.

Three Guard Blocks or Double Blocks and a Back Kick Combination

For this combination, your opponent should be a little slower than you. A back kick can only be possible if you have regained the momentum. You can only do that if you are quick enough.

To successfully do the combination, here are the scenarios and steps you should make.

1. Your opponent will throw a side kick or a roundhouse kick against you. You will block it using the guard block or double block. He will drop his leg in front of you or between your leg to keep the distance closer.

2. Take a step backward and stand in a back stance every time you block.

3. After your last block, quickly pivot your current front foot and do a back kick.

Below is an illustration to help you understand the steps.

Variation:

Instead of a back kick, you can throw a back fist instead. The back fist will be more unexpected and simpler.

To change the last steps into a back fist, on the third block, switch to a palm block. Hold the leg and pull your opponent closer. Then, pivot your front foot and throw a back fist with your rear hand.

Instead of a backfist, you can throw an uppercut or a combination of punches. You can also do the thrust knifehand strike or a regular knifehand strike on the neck.

You can also counter with a roundhouse, or a sidekick. Your opponent's body will be almost slanted away from you and a front kick may not be feasible.

Tips on how to defend yourself correctly

1.   Always strike with the aim to get away. The best way to defend yourself is to end the fight by running away. When a person is trying to attack you, he has the intention to harm you. The more you stay in the fight, you are putting yourself at a greater risk of being hurt. Thus, when your opponent is down, escape as fast as you can and call for help.

2.   Always make sure to hit the pressure points. The pressure points will cause pain and damage to your opponent. It will open an opportunity for you to leave the fight. The pressure point you should look for when counterattacking are the following:

- Head

- Temple

- Neck or throat

- Shoulder or the area near the clavicle

- Area just below the armpit

- Sternum or the middle part of the chest

- Solar plexus, which is the center point below the center of your ribs and above your abdomen.

- Ribs

- Instep

- Groin

3. Keep your focus. Do not let your temper or fear control you when someone is attacking you. If you become hot-tempered, you may end up staying in the fight to show your opponent what you can do. If you are terrified, you may not be able to correctly defend yourself.

Hence, keep your focus. Always tell yourself not to get hit. You should also encourage yourself to wait for the right time to hit your opponent. If you keep fighting, you will get tired and will have no power to run away when the opportunity arrives.

Chapter 7: Sport Poomsae

(By Instructor Mitch Wisner and Instructor Shannon Clousing)

Mitch and Shannon are key KAT black belts and instructors who began the KAT sport poomsae program when the form of competition was introduced by the WTF.

Sport poomsae is a new way of doing forms competitions that began in the last couple of years. It is open only to black belts and is a major departure from previous tradition in that the forms required are based on age rather than rank. It has resulted in the standardization of poomsae throughout the world in order to have everyone on a level, and equal playing field. Before this type of competition, every school had their own nuances that they added to their forms; whether it be various chambering methods, targeting, stances, or execution of specific technique.

With this new style of competition scoring will focus on two major areas. First is the accuracy of technique (start and finish point, chambering of blocks and strikes and detail). Second is presentation (speed, balance, motion, power and rhythm).

One of the most noticeable changes in Sport Poomsae is the stances. Many of them have been shortened. This was done to make the style more 'Korean' and distinct from the Japanese influence that Taekwondo carries from its early history. The international standard also helps eliminate referees being biased against certain techniques based on the way their masters have taught them.

It's a way for older competitors, who no longer spar, to be involved in the competition side of Taekwondo.

The competition itself is single elimination with a round robin system. If there are more than 18 competitors, they will start with a preliminary round of forms from the 1st Compulsory Group. If there are 17 or less competitors, they will use 2 forms from the 2nd Compulsory Group and choose the 8 highest scorers as finalists. Finally, if there are 8 competitors or less, they will proceed directly to the Final Round and pick the top 4 competitors. All poomsae should be completed within 1 to 2 minutes for all divisions, whether it is Individual, Team, or Pair competition.

Similar to sparring, Sport Poomsae is separated into divisions by age. They are:

- Cadet (age 10-13)

o 1st Compulsory: Taegeuk 2-5

o 2nd Compulsory: Taegeuk 6 - Koryo

- Juniors (age 14-18)

o 1st Compulsory: Taegeuk 4 - 7

o 2nd Compulsory: Taegeuk 8 - Taeback

- 1st Seniors (age 19-30), 2nd Seniors (age 31-40)

o 1st Compulsory: Taeguek 6 - Koryo

o 2nd Compulsory: Keumgang - Sipjin

- 1st Masters (age 41-50)

o 1st Compulsory: Taegeuk 8 - Taeback

o 2nd Compulsory: Pyongwon - Chonkwon

- 2nd Masters (age 51-60)

o 1st Compulsory: Koryo - Pyongwon

- o   2nd Compulsory: Sipjin - Hansu
- •   3rd Masters (age 60+)
- o   1st Compulsory: Koryo - Pyongwon
- o   2nd Compulsory: Sipjin - Hansu
- •   1st Team (age 15-35)
- o   1st Compulsory: Taegeuk 6 - Koryo
- o   2nd Compulsory: Keumgang - Sipjin
- •   2nd Team (age 36+)
- o   1st Compulsory: Taegeuk 8 - Taeback
- o   2nd Compulsory: Pyongwon - Chonkwon

Here is a progression of how a competition would go:

•Preliminary Round: Competitors will be asked to perform two of the four poomsae in their divisions 1st compulsory group. Only competitors with scores in the top half of their division will move onto the Semi-Final Round.

•Semi-Final Round: Competitors will be asked to perform two of the four poomsae in their divisions 2nd compulsory group. Only competitors with scores within the top 8 of their division will move onto the Final Round.

•Final Round: Competitors will be asked to perform two of the four poomsae in their divisions 2nd compulsory group. Of the eight competitors only the top four will place in either, 1st, 2nd, 3rd, or 3rd place.

In the event of a tie, the winner will be chosen based on the highest presentation score. If another tie exists, they will perform a final poomsae differing from the previous two they had just competed with. If there is still no clear winner, all scores from the competition will be compared to figure out the victor.

The scoring criteria for poomsae is rather strict. There are two categories that judges will look at. Each technique comes with a deduction of 0.1, or 0.5. If the competitor continues to make the same mistake on any technique, they will receive a maximum of 0.5 points deduction for that specific mistake.

- Technique
- Accuracy of Basic Movement
o Starting point

- Ending point
- Path of motion
- Hand/fist rotation
• Poomsae detail
- Movement progression
- Total movements associated with each combination
• Presentation
- Skills
  - [ ] Accuracy
  - [ ] Speed
  - [ ] Balance
• Expression
- Strength/speed/rhythm – does the form have good fluidity and less robotic?

There are several defined lines on the body where blocks end. For example, an out-to-in middle block ends right at the mid-line of the body. There is to be no "audible breathing" or "hissing" during the form. This is to further separate the style from ITF forms. People should also not announce their school name, or instructor's name. Unless otherwise specified, kicks will be to a specific target (the chest or face). The first choice is the face, but if that cannot be achieved, like for older age levels, the second choice will be chest. It is also very important to have the correct placement for hand techniques as well, including punches, elbow strikes, back fists, etc. Hands and feet should end the movement at the same time, as to "snap" into place. All blocks should be chambered with the blocking hand on the outside, and strikes with the striking hand on the inside.

Deductions will be either 0.1, or 0.5

- 0.1 Deductions
  - Incorrect motion
  - Poor balance
  - Foot angle in stance
  - Poor chambering
  - Poor foot recoil

- Blocking past midline of body
- Blocking with wrong arm
- Incorrect chambering for strikes
- Blocks and strikes at incorrect area.
- Kicking with wrong part of foot
- Wrapping hand around elbow on elbow strike
- Foot and hand do not end at the same time
- Hesitating
- Rhythm lacking
- Relaxation and tension should alternate well
- Flexibility and grace lacking
- Incorrect uniform
- Stance and Technique do not finish at the same time

- 0.5 Deductions

o Turning the wrong way

o Extremely poor balance

o No Kiyap

o Kiyap in the wrong place

o Incorrect stance/technique Added techniques or motions

o Missed techniques

o Stomping where there is none

o Not stomping where there should be

o Multiple of the same mistake will be capped at 0.5

o Repeating from the beginning

o Not ending within one foot length of your starting position

o Robotic performance

o Performing a move with the incorrect speed

o   Improper breathing

o   Eye focus doesn't go along with the current movement

o   Lack of fluency, flexibility, and power

Chapter 8: Sparring (Kyroogi)

Sparring Introduction

(With contributions from Master Tanya Paterno)

Master Tanya Paterno is a forth degree black belt and former MVP of Cornell Taekwondo who has won numerous medals at the Collegiate National Championships, US National Championships, and US Open, and was the first person to win four consecutive spots on the INCTL All Star Team. She is currently an instructor at Chung Ma's Taekwondo in New York.

Taekwondo sparring is an exciting form of competition. Although the fundamentals are simple, it takes many years of dedicated practice and conditioning to master them. What follows is not a comprehensive guide on how to spar, but some general tips that can come in handy in certain situations.

The basic point of sparring is to score more points than your opponent. Read through the full competition rules to understand how to play the game, especially as there are small changes every few years. Points come from either attacks or counter attacks. The natural stance, or sparring position, faces sideways. This leads to two basic positions in sparring, open stance and closed stance. In open stance, both competitors have their hogus facing the same direction. The name comes from the fact that both are open to a rear leg roundhouse kick. Closed stance is the opposite, where both hogus are facing in opposite directions. Knowing which stance you are in is important as certain techniques will work differently depending how your opponent is standing.

There are several kicks and exchanges that you must be familiar with. For example, from open stance, back kick counters roundhouse kick. From closed stance, back leg roundhouse kick counters back leg ax kick. You must drill these until they become like reflexes. Once you become proficient at the basics of attacking and counter attacking, you should start to add in trickery. Each match is a physical battle, but it is also a mental battle. You have to think and guess ahead at what your opponent is going to try to do. Similarly, you should try to lead your opponent in a certain way. Showing your kicks ahead of time by changing your position or shifting your weigh is called telegraphing. Look to see if your opponent is showing something. Usually this occurs in more inexperienced sparrers. Learn to hide your next movements. Clear your mind— if you don't know what you are going to do, your opponent won't either. At the same time, learn to intentionally show something in order to draw your opponent to react. This is called faking or trapping. The point of faking is to draw your opponent to counter, and then to recounter his counter. For instance, player A might notice that player B wants to throw a back kick. So player A might fake a roundhouse kick to the open side, and let player B throw his back kick. Then, player A might recounter with a roundhouse kick. However, to go one more level if the same thing happened again player B might fake that he was faked out, and when player A recounters with the roundhouse kick, player B might have the back kick ready again. Usually, there will be only 1 or 2 levels in the attacks and counter attack game, but at the most you should think three moves ahead.

Managing the time and the ring are also important. Always know how many rounds (3 or 2) you are sparring and how long they are. Do not be impatient and rush it to attack if the time is not right. Think through your attacks and what you are going to do. If you have four or six minutes to spar, don't become impatient and throw a match's worth of attacks in the first minute.

Most matches will have electronic scoring. In this case, you can see how both the time and the score are progressing throughout the match. If you are nearing the end of a match and know that you are ahead in points, you can protect your lead. You can wait for you opponent to attack, then counter. Do not sit dormant, but it is not urgent for you to attack to score. Be on the lookout for head shots, which are a fast way to make up points when time is short. Head shots are worth three points (since 2011 spinning head shots are worth 4 points) but are not allowed for all divisions. Generally only 14 and above black belts (and sometimes adult color belts) will be allowed full head contact. Others will be allowed no head contact (kids) or light head contact.

Always know where you are in the ring. Try not to be forced into a corner. This would be valuable to your opponent in that he now has two choices. He can attack you without you having the ability to move away, or he can force you out of bounds resulting in a penalty against you. If you find yourself caught in a corner it is important to know how to clinch and circle around, thereby getting out of the corner and maybe even forcing your opponent into the corner.

Punching is a valuable way to disrupt your opponent's flow of attack. This disruption might be short, but it is enough time for you to throw a kick or two and possibly score. Be sure that you punch, and don't push with an open hand. A punch can score a point if it is hard enough and clear enough.

When you are sparring, you will want to recognize if your opponent is taller or shorter than you are. If they are shorter than you are, it is in your advantage to be farther away from them. Therefore, you can be at a distance to score, but out of their range to hit you. If they are taller than you are, you should try to be closer, thereby again out of their range to score. One way of doing this is to clinch. Regardless of size, there is an 'idle position' where neither of you can score off the line. Learn how to recognize this distance.

Another important concept to understand is that of acceleration. Acceleration is defined as the change in velocity, which can either be speeding up or slowing down, or a change of direction. Constant speed can be timed easily, even if the speed is fast. In order to confuse your opponents, you must learn how to change your speed. A slow switch could cause your opponent to relax just enough that you can throw a fast roundhouse kick immediately afterwards and they might not have time to recover and then respond to your attack. Similarly, if you can move in directly on your opponent but then slide to the side at the last second, you may be able to cause him to counter your original motion and then you will be able to recounter successfully.

Taekwondo is currently changing rules with respect to things like the use of video replay, coach's challenge cards, and the use of electronic body protectors. With the electronic protectors, you kick your opponent and if it is hard enough (and contact is made with the sock) a point will automatically go up on the scoreboard. You will likely use several different ways when sparring in the dojang, sparring in local tournaments, or competing in the national championships. Since head shots have now become 3 points and points are scored for any contact, Olympic Taekwondo has started making much more use of the front leg and has become more similar to fencing.

Three Main Types of Techniques

Attacking - The first type of techniques developed were attacking techniques. On a low level of sparring, both players will attack each other and whoever attacks stronger will win.

Counterattacking – Soon, people started developing counterattacking techniques. This way, you can still defeat someone who is a better attacker than you by either avoiding his kick and coming back with your own or by counterattacking simultaneously.

Trapping – Once both players develop good counterattacks, the match can be very boring as both just stand there because neither wants to attack the other. This brought on the need for trapping techniques. The idea here is to call your partner to attack by 'making him an offer he can't refuse.' You then apply your counterattack. All traps must have an illusion of safety, a bait (cheese), and a hammer. In sparring, the bait is yourself, or the perceived ability to score on you and the hammer is your counterattack. It's important to note that traps can be defeated by speed. The worst thing is to set out a trap and have a fast mouse come in and take the cheese and escape before the hammer comes down. The more experienced your opponent is, the more likely it is that they will know you are trying to trap them, and the larger 'cheese' you will have to put in your trap.

In general, someone who attacks a lot will lose to someone who is patient and counterattacks, and someone who likes to do a lot of counterattacks will be defeated by someone with good trapping skills. In practice, a good competitor will need to be proficient at all three sets of skills.

Deceptive Motions (Faking)

Making deceptive motions is a very important part of Sport Taekwondo. In the black belt division, everyone has good technique. Everyone can kick hard and make a good strategy. How good they are at deceiving their opponent is one thing that separates the truly superior athletes. It is important to note that making deceptive motions should not be considered dishonorable, as long as it is within the rules. In fact, the ability to fool another skilled player is the mark of a great competitor. All deceptive motions have a few things in common. First of all, if you are faking a move, then your fake has to look like the beginning part of that move. The other thing to remember is that often a split second can make all the difference between success and failure. Thus if your fake can cause your partner to hesitate even that much, your attack will have a much higher chance of success. There are many types of deceptive motions that you may make in a match:

Fake an attack to draw out a counter – If your partner favors a certain counter attack, fake the related attack so that they can counter and then recounter their kick.

Fake a speed – Move at a slow speed for a few seconds so that your partner is lulled by your slower speed and then explode at a fast speed. Conversely, move very fast and then suddenly go slow. You may be able to catch them off rhythm.

Fake a direction – Get your partner to think you are moving one way and then switch quickly to take advantage.

Fake a mistake – Pretend to look at the scoreboard, slip, or be distracted. Then when he tries to attack you, have your counter ready.

Fake being faked out – It sounds a bit complicated, but when they do a fake, pretend that you fell for it, while being ready to recounter their counter.

Fake a strategy – The most common time this occurs is when you want to counterattack, for instance if you are winning and the time is running down. If your partner knows that he doesn't have to worry about your attack, his own attack will be more successful. Thus, keep making aggressive attacking motions and do one or two attacks to keep your partner's mind thinking of many things at once.

Check – This is not so much a fake, but you will stomp hard on the floor with your front leg while moving your body forward as if attacking. Checks can sometimes show you what your opponent was planning to do by how they move their body. It's a good idea to use checks before you attack because at the very least you can disrupt your opponent's rhythm.

Deceptive Telegraphing – This is an advanced technique where you can drop subtle hints to show you partner what you are planning to do. However, you show him things that you are not planning to do with the intention of leading him into a trap.

Psychology of Selection

Scientific studies show that reaction time increases based on the number of things that you are thinking about at one time.

For instance, imagine that you are sparring and you know that your partner is going to do one of two things (i.e., either attack the closed side or open side.) You have to mentally prepare a counter for both. If you wait to see what he is doing, then make a decision, then perform the counterattack, you have, say, a 50% chance of guessing correctly. However, if you have one counter in your head and prepare for it, and go for that one unless the other one comes, you may increase your chance of success. Say you have a 90% chance of a successful counter if you guess right, and a 40% chance if you guess wrong and have to adapt. Assuming that your partner has a 50% chance of throwing either technique, now you have a 65% chance of scoring.

In any case, the fewer things that you have to think about, the faster your reaction time will be. Thus, in sparring it's important to clear your mind and focus on just a few trains of thought. The more things that you can force your opponent to think about, the slower his reaction time will be.

Sparring Stance

Master Matthew Bailey is a 5th degree black belt and has been with the KAT for most of his life. He formerly served in the US Air Force and represented the United States Armed Forces in Taekwondo at the World Military Championships.

A proper sparring stance refers to the body position that provides any technical or tactical advantage to the opponent. Every move is made from this position. The most important thing to consider is what is the most effective position? It is a difficult question because there isn't specific stance that is suitable for all athletes. It will vary based on the individual's particulars such as attitude, mood, and the strategy. While it's not essential to create a definitive policy there are some fundamental principles:

The space between feet shouldn't be too wide at all, it should be about shoulder width from each other.

The body should be flexible and fluid so that it can spring off of the feet to move quickly, while maintaining balance.

By slightly bending your knees, the weight of the leading leg will facilitate faster moving.

The shoulders should be free with arms that are not contracted so that you can move quickly.

A more extended stance will make a bigger space between yourself and the opponent. This can also provide greater power when you perform moves such as a speedy kicks. But, it can also lower your head.

Make sure you don't signalize your kicks with the way you hold your body.

Charles's Sparring Tips on Sparring:

(By Charles DeGuzman)

Charles DeGuzman holds a third degree black belt, and one of the KAT's most elite students. He helped develop advanced kicks, and was among the first students to perform the hook kick in 540, and won the national championship on board breaking it.

While sparring, it's crucial to be able to assess your opponent's strengths and weaknesses However, prior to competition you must be able to employ a variety of strategies in the arena. As an example, for instance, it is important to know that you can't simply walk in and use a specific footwork or kick. Techniques for sparring in competition are divided into three types. There are circular kicks (roundhouse and hook kick). They are referred to as circular as they always strike your opponent on the opposite side, and they require strong snapping motion. Another type of kick is linear kicks (side or push as well as the back kick). They are linear since they are always straight and often times rely on the body's weight instead of snapping. The last are the strikes (jab or reverse punches). They are seldom employed for fighting. They are usually employed to make a space between you and your opponent to allow your kicks when you are you are countering. It is essential to have at the very least 1 kick for each group, since they will quickly counter one another. You ought to know how to punch. The more you are aware the more you are able to make your opponent think twice, but you only have to a certain point. fancy techniques such as butterflies or 540 kicks twists can cause you to lose points due to simple counters, or put you at risk. Kicks are used for a reason at the right moment, not to are attractive. You must also be aware of the positions you should use. The distance between your feet will give you the fastest attacks. A half and one shoulder widths give you acceleration and some strength. Two shoulder widths give you the strongest attacks. The stances you take will vary depending on the situation. If you're in a long distance from the clinch, you may opt for the wide stance for the initial strike however, you should switch to a an angled shoulder stance as you are close to the point of clinching.

What are the best ways to study your opponent? The first step is to understand the little details such as which foot is always facing forward whether he is left or right-footed or does he engage in combat or defensively? What length are his legs as compared to yours, is he keeping his hands in a downward position or do they prefer to stand either in a closed or open stance or closed stance, what's his favourite kick, and how does he react when you try to fake. These little details can be very helpful in deciding on the best strategy. You can profit from his mistakes, or even counter his strategies. The next step is more technically-oriented. What happens if I make this or kick in a specific place, like closed or open or even from the clinch? Risking your life can aid in studying your opponent, however you must remain aware of implications.

So what do you do next? After you've gathered the details of your foe, you are able to apply them to your tactics and use to beat him. For example when he responds to a round kick by using an back kick, I'd perform a roundhouse motion feint before countering that back kick. Here are some tactics to apply against various types of opponents.

"He's bigger than You." This happens at least once during your career of sparring. This implies that he's got longer legs than you when playing an activity that requires the use of long legs. The first thing to remember is to keep your hands on the ground! If you kick your head, it could be an arm kick for him. In addition, you should be careful not to step on him. The longer the legsare, the more difficult to get him back for another attack after having missed. Thirdly, remain inside. If you stay close to the enemy, you stop his attack , and at same time, you close your gap, which causes him to withdraw or to jump back. It's much easier to strike forwards rather than back. Again keep your hands up. Then you are in his high attack area. Make a fake move and then go in. Then, make him kick the ball not miss you, and then go.

"He's Shorter." This is basically the exact opposite of the tall approach. It is recommended to employ many cut fakes and kicks. The key is to stay away. If he does come into the room, you must cut him off using the linear kick (cutting side kicks are the most effective) then move to the side and strike. After you have cut off his back, he will not cease to attack. He could take a step back and then launch the roundhouse. If you back step to keep your distance exactly as you want to in order to counter. If you're quick enough and speed, you may at times take them out by using an axe, back kick, or high roundhouse, while bouncing back.

"He's Too aggressive." If your opponent is a fan of attack, allow him to for an extended period of time, but you must keep sliding or clinching. It is possible to counter immediately after the sidestep, and then make a clinch. Utilize your reverse kick to throw him off his balance. Make sure he isn't wasting energy and wasting his points. Make use of a variety of fakes to keep him frightened and moving. Someone who is too aggressive tends to be standing on one leg. You can knock him off balance by using a the linear attack and counter when the attacker is fighting. Rememberthat the majority of points come caused by counters.

"He waits a Lot as well as Counters." These kinds of players tend to be the most intelligent. One thing you do not intend to commit is engage in a violent attack with carelessness. Also it is the fakes that are the most important element. If they are waiting and then respond, you must create fakes that are convincing because they are aware that they'll be coming. When you make the feint, be prepared for counters. If he fails to hit the counter, it's now your turn. Utilize your own strategy against him, and then clinch.

"This Guy's Fast." If you're competing against someone who's quick then you shouldn't be able to compete in a speed race. You'll be beaten. It is best to strike when his leg is up in the air. The time needed to lower his leg down and strike a second time should be the same length or more than the time you throw your strike. It is important to force him to throw that kick so that he throws your own. How? Tricks and flimsies.

"This Guy is a Heavyweight or something!" This is your issue! You ought to have considered losing weight prior to entering the race.

A skilled sparer is quick and clever, able to adapt to any situation and defeat his adversaries; he should first be able to conquer his physical and mental limitations however. Don't be afraid to risk your life in the boxing ring. Never be scared to use your kicks or take on opponents. Always remain calm, calm confident, and at ease. Everyone is skilled in the world of elite competition. It's the mind that separates the first and second.

Video Analysis

Recording your sparring games and techniques is an crucial part of your practice. When you are in a sparring match things occur in a matter of seconds. The players and coaches are taught to be able to spot their opponents however, with all the adrenaline pumping and the restricted time and distance it is inevitable to overlook some thing.

Tape study is an excellent method to improve your abilities. But you must be aware of the right way to tape it and how to do it. At at a minimum, record all your matches. If you're able to then, you must record the matches of every player who is in the same division. Even if you don't fight against them all but you could spar with them in the future. It is also possible to observe how they respond in various situations. If you're not black belt, you must film black belt match.

What should you be looking for in your tapes? It is necessary to watch them over and over to be able to comprehend all of the information. In the beginning, you should look for major lesson, i.e., things that are easily apparent. You'll discover a lot about the strategies that worked or did not work, as well as major strategic mistakes or the correct choices you made. But, you must examine the details of your adversaries and conduct a statistical analysis of them. Check if they favor open or closed stances and also which leg they prefer.

Complete the table below by putting a tick mark each time an opponent makes some of the kicks listed below.

Attack Right is attacked Left Countered Right Left

Closed Stance

Open Stance

If you are looking at your own technique, search at the technical precision. This should be done frame-by-frame, in slow movement. If the technique didn't work check out the reason. For example do you think your back kick not work because you weren't reacting in a timely manner, or was the trajectory of your leg too long? If it worked then note the reason why it did succeed.

Take note of the deceitful actions your opponents use and then look for patterns. Do they always double check twice before striking? Do they always try to fake the open side before striking on the side closed? Do they consistently pretend to be in the same spot in which they attack? In most cases, you'll detect patterns that your opponents do not even realize about. Of course, knowing that you need to conduct the same analysis for yourself to ensure that you don't get caught in the same pattern. Of course you will not likely repeat the same pattern each time however, If they do it more than at least 80 percent or 90 percent of the times, you can count on it to gain the advantage when you play them in the next game. Find 'tells' within their tactics, i.e., small variations in the way their fakes appear and their kicks appear.

Additionally, you should look for clues like what the coach is saying or the motions are made by him and the player is doing. Watch how the player reacts when they're losing points, or observe how they safeguard their advantage. If there are just five seconds remaining and they only have one shot to score, what kick is he going to attempt? And what is the best way to make it happen?

You can also look at how the other players react when the opponent or you earns one point. Find out what causes your opponent to be unhappy. In the event that your adversary is tough and you haven't had many opponents beating him, locate an opponent who has been successful and research the way they beat them. You might be able to employ a similar method.

Distance

AKA the "Donut Of Danger"

Taekwondo is often referred to as "a game of distance. In reality an extra inch can mean an important difference in the outcome between massive hit and a complete failure. However, how can your actual distance of striking be calculated, visualized and then extended?

An easy geometric estimate of distance that you can hit can be created by putting on one leg while turning one leg about the joint of your hip. The furthest point you'll be in a position to hit is at the hip level. If you lift your leg in order to hit higher, you'll reduce the distance of your kick. This means that you'll be able hit your opponent further from a distance if you hit them with your hip. The shape of the torus is called a torus however, it is often referred to as donut.

We'll reduce the analysis to two dimensions . We will then use a bird's eye perspective from the top looking down at both competitors. The following diagram shows the best competitor as well as his strike distance. It is important to note that the edges must be blurred so that a player isn't capable of delivering maximum power at the very limit the range. Inside dots depict the physique of the opponent, i.e., if any area within the blue circle comes into contact with the red dot, the blue player has the ability to score against that red participant. In this example both players are in a stalemate because neither of them can hit each other. The blue one is larger and has more distance (bigger circle) however, it is more in a position to strike from both sides (smaller outer circle).

Two players at a slack distance

The most common thing that happens during an actual sparring match can be seen in that the players move to a point at which they can easily hit the opponent typically the flurry distance. This is where both players can hit each other with ease. In this case, the player who is quicker is likely to earn more points, however the other player will take serious punishment if another player is more powerful. If one player is quicker and more powerful, the other player will have a chance to win in the long run, as long as he does not remain within the opponent's ideal distance.

Flurry distance is the distance at which each player is capable of hitting one another

It's evident the two options to stop an opponent's kick by moving back or moving forward. The white space shown in the images is the place that neither player can strike. Most often, one of the players will close the distance, and then end in an uninvolved clinch position. Clinching is an effective technique to deter the opponent who is quicker or to delay the game.

The the clinch position. The chests of the players are in contact, and neither is able to strike the other.

To gain the advantage in the game, one of the players must ensure that the game is played at his ideal distance. The distance is dependent on the player who has a greater distance.

Optimal Distance. The ideal distance differs for taller blue (left) in comparison to the smaller red (right)

If there's an increase in distance it is at a point at which you will be able strike your opponent, but he will not strike you. It is typically in the outer or inner the edge that you are able to reach. In the left half of the image the blue player places himself on the outside of his range. He's in a position to strike the red player, whereas the player in red is far away to strike back. In the right-hand side the red player moves inside and can strike the blue player however, the blue participant is far too near to hit the player efficiently. This is a reason for each participant to ask two fundamental questions:

1. How can I increase my "donut of risk"? It is important to increase your effective strike distance both outwards and inwards. The only method to achieve it is by practicing striking the targets further to each other, and further more. The kicks vary when distance increases. They are great for the inside and roundhouse kicks work well to increase distance. Additionally, the torus was drawn using the hip as the same location in space. With a hip movement, you can move the entire torus direction. For example, if you want to strike in a clinch, pull your hips inwards and you'll be able to hit more closely to your body.

2. How do I keep the game at my ideal distance? The answer is simple: you should have a great footwork. You should be able to reach the desired location and then counter opponent's moves. If, for instance, you are at your ideal distance, and your opponent moves forward, you have to reverse to keep the distance same. Also, you must be able to move

laterally or diagonally to cut distance swiftly. The person with the greater range is naturally in the lead since the player who is shorter will hit his target prior to the distance of the shorter player.

Concepts of the future

A deceitful RangeDeceptive Range - None of the strategies discussed here is hidden and the strategies are well-known. But the edges of danger vary for every participant. If you can reach greater distance than your opponent would expect, you could be able get to your ideal distance even though your opponent thinks that you're in a stale position. Then you'll be able to hit and surprise the opponent.

Drawing out kicksThere is a brief moment of safety following a kick from your adversary. This is the perfect time for a player who is smaller (red) to be in the donut of risk of the larger player (blue). Red may inch in blue's maximum distance and cause blue to attack. Red is then able to slide back and dodges the kick, after that, it rushes into strike and bring the match to the red's ideal distance.

Expanding Range with Steps While every time an athlete steps up to donuts move however, if the player takes a step and strikes instantly it is possible to increase his range. This is the case for kicks like hop roundhouse kicks with back legs and double kicks.

Let the opponent close distance- Sometimes it's in the favor of the shorter player to allow the taller player get closer and then challenge him. This may reduce the taller player's range advantage. This is why a back kicks are especially important for smaller players since they are unable to take on roundhouse kicks off the line against taller players. Because the taller player is already in the game and the smaller player is able to utilize his back kick to score without worrying over the height advantage that the taller one has. But, when playing with a back kick the shorter player is susceptible to being fucked to the larger player, and defeated when he finishes his spin.

But, it is important to be aware that the player who has shorter reach may be able to reduce in on the space, kick and clinch if substantially faster than larger players. This is only true in the event that the taller player not proficient at the pada chagie as well as receiving the kick. If the taller person slides backwards when throwing this kick, it will stop the shorter player from closing sufficiently.

Table of counterattacks and attacks

Unless otherwise stated the kicks must be done by kicking your back foot.

Closed Stance Techniques

Attack Counter Recounter

Roundhouse Roundhouse Back Kick

Roundhouse Front leg 360 degrees Back Hook or Kick

Roundhouse Cover Punch

Front leg Roundhouse back kick or the Spin Hook Kick Roundhouse

The Ax-Kick Roundhouse Kick Back Kick

Butterfly Kick Kick back Kick Spin Hook Kick

Side Kick or Push Roundhouse Back Kick

Open Stance Techniques

Attack Counter Recounter

Roundhouse Back Kick Roundhouse

Roundhouse Spin Hook Kick Roundhouse

Roundhouse Front Butterfly kick Back Kick

The Ax Kick Back Kick Spin Hook Kick Roundhouse

Ax Kick Double kick Double Kicks

Side Kicks or Pushes. A. Roundhouse Back Kick

360 back or hook kick Roundhouse Back Kick

Double kicks are particularly effective due to the fact that they strike both sides and are utilized to block almost any method, even double kicks. Furthermore, they are able to block and stop any counter attack that your opponent has devised. For example, if your opponent is countering with roundhouse kick, move into one side at first in order to end the attack. If he prefers to counter with a back kicks, move towards the closed side first.

Chapter 9: Weapons

Training in weapons isn't one of the primary elements that the majority of Taekwondo schools employ. But, the practice of traditional weapons is of great worth to any martial artist because of a number of reasons:

* Weapons may give an advantage to a weaker, smaller or disabled individual.

The underlying principles of the unarmed and armed fights are similar, weapons training will help you comprehend the techniques you use without weapons at a deeper level.

* Training in weapons is a significant cultural and social component of our heritage of martial arts.

All Weapons

Safety

Before we continue the training, a word of caution is needed. To train safely and effectively using weapons, your conduct must be more rigorous than the norm. Training with weapons, including simple, wooden, or cushioned ones, can be very risky. There is a chance to cause harm to yourself or others. This is why the practice of training with weapons was considered to be sacred in a variety of cultures. Here are some things to be aware of:

Always ensure that you practice in a clean space.

* Ensure that your weapon is safe and in good condition. The worst thing you could have is your weapon breaking and then part of it to be thrown at your friend.

* Learn difficult or obscure techniques using padded weapons before.

Do not do any contact training using sharp weapons.

Basics

In contrast to unarmed combat guns add a variety of ways to train. For example, we have the armed and unarmed. unarmed combat , and the battle between armed and. Armed. There are a variety of weapons to fight with. If it's swords against. spear? Or Bo vs. nunchuks? Naginata or. fan? How can we learn techniques that can aid us in all possible situations? Weapons that projectile (stars blowgun, bow and bows) are an entirely separate category and will be treated differently in the future. Our school has devised the following methods to teach firearms techniques.

However, with a few exceptions The weapon used to strike does not matter as much as the direction in which you strike. This applies to both defense and attack. Whatever weapon you're using you're always trying to strike with a certain level of precision which target critical areas.

Our school has developed the ten most basic strikes that are shown in the photo below. In the 9 strike, it is straightforward thrusting strike, and it is also a strike that strikes the hands of the opponent.

Each strike is also accompanied by an accompanying block. For example, a 3 strike made with any weapon can be protected by a 3-block using any weapon. Be aware that angle has precedence over the object. For example the straight strike that goes to the left of the neck is an high 4 strike, not two strikes.

Historically, weapons weren't taught differently to people with left hands. The reason for this is that the opposing force (3,5,7) will be performed similar to a striking technique (2,4,6) for the left handed person or. the right-handed person. The exact method is reversed. For example, a right handed person can perform a 3 strike using the same technique the same way a left-handed person is able to do a two strike.

After each weapon has these basic attack and block techniques, it is must complete some other fundamental protocol strategies. For instance, every weapon has to be equipped with a grip, an eye stance, a prepared position, and an option to return to a ready posture.

Each weapon could have additional methods and strikes that are unique to the weapon. For example the sword comes with drawing sheathing, disarming as well as cleaning methods. It could also feature special moves like spins release, figure 8s, spins role, fakes and more.

Each weapon needs the base form. It is essentially repeated moves in a specific sequence to aid in learning these moves. Some of the basic forms can be practiced with your partner.

The next step is that most weapons include a partner-form. This is actually two distinct forms, which when combined with a companion will create an exciting fight scene. Be careful to avoid hitting your partner.

Additionally, each weapon will come with one or more competition forms. These forms can be utilized directly in weapon form competitions and include several more impressive moves. Contrary to others, these forms can be customized and customized to suit the participant.

Sword

History: Swords were an integral part of almost every human civilization since the Bronze Age. They come in various dimensions and shapes. The most common sword we use is the curving Japanese style long sword. It is also known as the Katana, Tachi, or even a'samurai sword." The art associated using cutting, drawing and using this type of sword is commonly referred to as Iaido.

Kendo literally means "The way of swords" is a form of martial arts that is associated with sword training. It is a similar Korean martial art called Headong Gumdo. This style of fighting incorporates more inventive moves, such as kicks and spins. We will incorporate techniques from both disciplines at KAT.

Types:

Katana They are the razor-sharp, curving medal blades that are legendary. They've been used in Japan for centuries. But their use in the modern world is unlikely due to the risk involved in using the swords. Modern production lines Katana are generally made from only one piece of metal poured into the form of a mold. However, traditional high-quality swords are made of two separate pieces of steel. One is sturdy but will not have the ability to hold edge while the other one can be sharpened, but is brittle. The swordsmith would combine the first metal with the other, and it creates an axe that is sturdy and sharp.

Bokken They are wood replicas of the katanas. The traditional Samurai boy would be given the bokken upon his fifth birthday, and then begin his education. These swords are fantastic to use for forms training however they are not safe to be used on a person even with armor.

Shinai They are straight swords that are made of four pieces of bamboo. Their straightness is an issue for those who want to master curly swords, since they fall apart upon contact, they absorb the most part of the power of an hit. Therefore, Kendo is a form of combat. Kendo allows two opponents to attack each other using Shinai, as long as both are wearing complete protection (bogu.) Shinai also come with the yellow string. The string represents that the reverse that of the edge cutting.

The fitting: Kendo competition rules proscribe the weight and size of a shinai according to your age athlete. But, a reasonable estimate is that, if you put the shinai's point onto the flooring, the top of your tsuka (handle) will be raised toward your sternum.

Grip: A proper grip on the blade is vital to ensure that power is evenly distributed across the blade. In general, you should to hold your right hand close to the guard (tusba) as well as your left at the handle's base. The hands should be as close to each other as you can, since this will allow you to direct energy across the blade. In general your right hand acts as a guide , while the pulling motion of your left hand will perform majority of the task.

Attention Stance: When in the focus stance the sword is placed on the left end. This is accomplished by putting the sword on your belt or scabbard or holding the sword in your left hand.

Bow: The traditional bow is achieved by bringing the right hand over the heart using an upward push when bowing. There is an additional bow that sits, known as sankyo that is commonly used in the kendo.

Ready Stance: The position is also called Chudan or kamae. Your feet are laid out in a walking stance and the heel part of your rear leg elevated above the floor. The left arm is in line with your belt and the point of the sword is aimed towards the eyes of your opponent.

Fundamental Form fundamental form is a form for partners in which two players face one another. One of them leads by striking 1-9 as they move forward. While the other one counters with blocks 1-9 while going backwards. After the 9th block the blocker will respond with 9 strikes (tsuki strike).

Parter Forms: There's ten partner forms in Kendo that were created in the early 1900s. Seven of these forms use the longer blade (tachi) as well as three using shorter swords (kodachi). These 10 forms have been mastered by a black 1st degree belt from Kendo.

Contest Forms: The initial demo/competition form is the companion form of Demo Team.

The following form for competition is the 3rd Degree black belt form , which is from Headong Gumdo.

Techniques to use: There's a variety of sword tricks to choose from, including spinning and release.

Specific Techniques: The special methods that are used by swords include drawing, cutting, and sheathing methods.

Methods for Cleaning Blades (Chiburi) Also, swords require cleaning method for blades called Chiburi. When a sword is cut, cuts the swordsman has to clean the blade prior to when it can be put back in its scabbard. Otherwise, the scabbard could be difficult to wash. Most of the time, it's just one quick movement with the hand to clean blood and dirt out of the blade. When a fight was over and the battle was over, elaborate cleaning procedures were followed.

Nunchuks

History The entry on Wikipedia for the Nunchuks says:

While the exact source of the nunchaku isn't known the possibility is that it was created in

Okinawa. It is believed that the nunchaku was initially a flail with a shorter length that was employed to thresh rice (separate the grain from the husk). But some believe that this weapon wasn't created as a grain flail and was invented by a master of martial arts looking for a way to shield his personnel from the oppressive current government which is why he decided to break it into three parts. The three-sectioned weapon is known as the Sansetsukon. The nunchaku is derived from this, and then grew evolving into what it is today.

The weapon's creation is believed to have been a result of the ban on edged weapons under the Satsuma daimyo, due to their strict policy on controlling weapons after the invasion of Okinawa during the late 17th century. (Some believe it was likely to have been designed and made for this purpose, because the design of actual flails and pieces is too heavy to use for weapons and the fact that farmers from the peasantry weren't likely to be trained for combat improvised to professionals.) The modern nunchaku was modified to make it suitable for use as a weapon, and could be a relatively useless rice flail.

Different types: Nunchuks are available in a variety of kinds. The staves are made from wood (rattan bamboo, cherry,) or more recently , plastic and aluminum. The chain linking them could be either a chain link or string joined by ball bearings. Additionally, in the modern age, the ends may be designed to accommodate glowsticks or electronic lights.

Fitting the size of the piece ought to roughly equal the size of the forearm. The chain should be positioned by hanging the nunchuks across the sides of your hand, with your palm facing downwards. Both ends should be downwards, without any additional chain.

Nunchuk grip: They need to be securely held with one hand. A grip close to the chain will provide you with maximum control and a limited distance, while an end-to-end grip will provide you with the least control and the most range. Therefore, you might have to switch grips in a form or fight.

Attention Stance In the attention stance , you hold the nunchuks with your left hand and perform the normal attention stance.

Bow: Hold Nunchuks to your left. You can also make a Bow by placing the right hand over your heart.

Stand Ready: A position is just like an ordinary stance but you only hold the other end of each nunchuk within each palm.

Tricks: Tricks using nunchuks require spins hands, hand switches and chain-related techniques.

Bo Staff

The Bo staff has a long history. Bo staff is among the most ancient and flexible weapons. Since the time that a caveman killed another by a downed tree branch, mankind has utilized and improved the Bo staff.

Types: The majority of staffs are constructed from the length of a thin chunk of timber. They can also be constructed out of plastic, metal or even foam. Some staffs have a taper towards the end. They're designed for speedy spinning but aren't useful against another weapon. Staffs could also have a thing on the other end that isn't mop, broom or spear. The KAT staff methods are taught to ensure they can work with spears too.

Fitting: The rule of thumb is that staffs must be at least a couple of inches higher than the user, and up to 6 feet tall.

Grip: The staff can be held in a variety of ways The most popular method is to hold it in a way that your hands divide it into three parts. The hands in the front are looking up with palms upwards and the reverse hand will be facing the palm down.

Attention Stance The attention stance is using the staff in the left hand, and pulled out away from your body in a 45-degree angle.

Bow: When bowing using the staff, allow it to extend toward the left at 45 degrees , then raise your right hand toward your chest.

Ready Stance: In the prepared posture, you place your right foot facing forward and the staff is in the grip mentioned above.

Special Techniques and Tricks: Special techniques and tricks include spins, block-to-strike combinations, as well as aerial moves using the staff.

Chapter 10: Demonstration Techniques

(Trick Kicks)

Demonstration techniques are techniques which look stunning, but they aren't likely to perform in a real match or fight. Demonstration techniques aren't mandatory in the school curriculum however they can be beneficial to master because they are engaging, stimulating and help learn concepts that are used in routine methods.

But, these demonstration methods could be risky if not taught correctly. They are often higher in speed, are faster, and can be more inverted than regular methods. Additionally, there aren't enough trained instructors for demonstration techniques. Make sure you have the right instructors and pads for trying out the latest demo strategies. We've created the following step-by-step guides for you to learn a few of the most common demonstration techniques.

This guide covers the fundamentals. Watch the videos of the methods.

The first path is Z as well as X Axis Spinning Techniques.

1. Basics - You must first master the basics of kicks such as the spin hook or roundhouse.

2. Reverse Step, Roundhouse You'll kick with the front foot following the reverse step.

3. Butterfly kick - A butterfly kick is when you jump just before you kick. This is also referred to as 360 Roundhouse.

4. Raize - It's similar to the butterfly kick, but there's no kick. The goal is to go as high as you can.

5. A 540-degree kick. Next step, execute the butterfly kick, and then kick the foot that is landing on the kicking foot.

6. Swipe to the right - This move is one that's 540 the point where your body turns in the X direction instead of the Z axis.

7. A 540-degree Hook Kick You can now use the foot that didn't hit the ground and kick a hook using it.

8. You can now do 720 kicks. you are able to complete any of these by modifying or using multiple kicks.

Path 2: Y Axis Spinning Techniques

1. Kung Fu Butterfly Kick - In this kick, you'll begin by doing an opposite step, and then jump up, keeping your chest in line with the floor. Then you will be landing on the foot from which you took off (180 vertical spin)

2. Butterfly Twist - Now , you will be landing on the foot you took off with. It's crucial to leap high and spin swiftly. (360 vertical spin)

3. Hypertwist - This time , you return to the beginning landing on the other foot that you started using. (540 vertical spin)

4. Corkscrew Twist: Bring your leg like you're trying to do an upwards kick. Then, leap and twist up in the air. (360 air spin)

3rd Path: Forwards Tumbling

1. Front Roll

2. Diving Roll: Try going over more and more obstacles. Be sure to turn your body diagonally to 45 degrees, and spread the force of your fall.

3. Front Flip TuckNow, you'll flip and move across the floor from foot to foot. Be sure to tighten the tuck. When you use a sword, it transforms into The JumpSlash of Ninja Gaiden.

4. Brandi A front-facing flip, with an inverse turn.

5. Webster - This starts with an ax kick and then you apply the force to lift your body up enough so that you can flip.

Chapter 11: Bruce Lee's Combat Principles

In this chapter, we'll examine the initial fundamentals of combat of Jeet Kune Do as taught by Bruce Lee. Certain combat rules in JKD require more detail, so they'll be covered in subsequent chapters.

Bruce Lee believed that these fundamental principles of fighting are evident and you'll eventually discover the truth as you learn and master martial arts. If you are looking to prove their validity and authenticity, all you have to do is practice these principles.

MMA Proves JKD Principles

It's important to remember the fact that MMA has already proven to be valid at the very least one of these concepts of fighting. In other words, the many years of training and experience that have been accumulated in the field in mixed martial arts has given a stamp of approval for Lee's methods and specifically on the four areas of combat.

In reality, the stages of combat that are described in MMA are precisely the same as what Lee calls ranges. To become a skilled fighter, you must master the art of striking (punch or elbow, kick and knee) grappling, takedowns as well as take down defense submission methods, clinch fighting and so on.

All-Martial Artist = A Well-Rounded Fighter

Since the time that were UFC 1 to 3, everybody has noticed that the fighters who have only learned to stand-up or simply grappling on the ground will not get to the top of the fight. It is not necessary to concentrate on everything. Actually, you could learn one or two of them and be able to remain effective in other fields.

It is important that you are well-rounded. Learn the most efficient, effective and beneficial aspects of each martial art. There is no need to fuss with the techniques you don't utilize. The ability to master every technique isn't essential, but effectiveness is. Bruce Lee once said:

"I do not fear the person who has tried 10,000 kicks a time however I am afraid of the one who has practiced just one kick 10,000 times."

The Intercepting Fist

In addition, Bruce Lee has also been famously quoted as saying that "the most effective defense is an effective offensive." It is where the concept of interception is applied. This is why the concept that of "intercepting fist" gives evidence of self-defense. A preemptive attack is definitely effective in all real-life circumstances. It can be used even for those who are weaker or smaller or are at a disadvantage physically.

Many things could be "intercepted" and not only kicks, punches or attempts to take down. The non-verbal and verbal signals coming from your opponent may signal his intention and his future actions - so you should be able to take advantage of the situation and respond with an appropriate and decisive response.

One Last Note

Before getting into the real fighting rules which Bruce Lee taught, it must be noted Bruce Lee also taught that one should:

"Obey the rules, but not be legally bound by them"

Learn all you can about everything you have to know. Learn from the information that is in the book. Take the information you find helpful to you. Remember that you're not tied to what you've acquired simply because you'll be constantly learning. Make sure you are flexible in your experiences of life and fight. The rules you discover will allow you to swing as a tree branch. the tree. You are the only thing that matters. Your ever developing self must be in control. Bruce Lee also once said:

"Notice that the most rigid tree is the easiest to break and the willow or bamboo can be able to withstand twisting with the winds."

When you are learning these basic combat strategies, you must effectively be the bamboo to learn to read the winds (the fundamentals of combat) and bend to them, follow the rules, but remember that you're the person who ultimately decides which actions to take. You're the one in charge and you're who is in charge.

Principle 1 - The Straight Lead

This is among the very first concepts that will learnt by students in JKD. It simply means that you position the dominant hand in front to lead your hand. This is different from the traditional approach of boxing, where your dominant hand is held behind and you are leading with you finger (the not-dominant hand).

Boxers typically use many jabs. they usually have small power and are utilized to prepare the next punches in combination. A straight punch instead of a jab using your dominant hand is the basis of your attack in JKD.

Similar to the jab, it can be used to set up the other attacks. However, your lead attack will be powerful, fast and much more precise. It is important to note that lead straight isn't one that can be considered a power strike, it is more of an a speed strike. If you're right-handed then you must have your right hand slightly extended towards your opponent.

The hand should be relaxed and do not strain your muscles on the right hand. If you hit your opponent and strike, you'll only tighten your fist, and contract your muscles when you hit. Since your hand is slightly extended and directed towards your opponent, it will get to the target faster. Because this punch is fired from the center of your body this makes it more precise.

This is by far the most powerful and most precise punch in JKD. Although it is hit at a central point, it is possible to throw it at various angles to make it more dynamic.

Principle #2 - Be Like Water

This is not just a rule that applies to fighting , but to the world of everyday life too. Bruce Lee often times emphasized the importance of fluidity. You can't be rigid. It is essential to be able to change your approach to the situation and the ever-changing times. A method, strategy or method may have worked previously, however if it's not working for the current issue or opposition Then you must be able to develop new strategies and solutions to achieve success.

Bruce Lee once said the following on The Pierre Barton Show in 1966:

"Empty your mind. Be in shapeless and formless water. If you put water in the cup, it transforms into the cup. Put water in the bottle, and it turns into the bottle. If you put it into a teapot and it transforms into the teapot. The water will flow or it may fall. Be water, my friend."

In that way, in your daily life as well as in martial arts, you must be able to adjust to different circumstances. You must be able to perform regardless of the circumstances you might be confronted with. Punch when you need to punch and kick when you need to kick, and grapple whenever you have to and do whatever is needed in the event of needing it. This way, you'll always be open to learning new things and information. In that sense , the jeet-kune do instructor is constantly developing.

Chapter 12: Combat Principles

Principle #3 - Attacks that are not Telegraphed and Moving

This is not just a rule of thumb to fights, but to the world of. Bruce Lee often times When someone is preparing to punch , you can anticipate the most powerful punch to be coming at you. This is the same for every attack. There are signals of movement, expressions, and involuntary queues which will reveal your opponent's identity, making it clear what his next move will be.

Telegraphed attacks can be prevented and countered. This is the reason JKD practitioners do not use these types of attacks. Non-telegraphed and explosive attacks are preferred in this art of fighting. If a punch is not telegraphed, it is likely to leave your opponent in the dark.

You'll catch your opponent off guard. With the initial surprise attack, your opponent will be left to guess the direction that your subsequent strike is coming from, which is an advantage, especially in real-life situations where one strike could mean the difference between life or death.

According to Lee Lee, is to just to let your arms move freely. Make sure you don't make any wind-up movements prior to you strike. The same principle applies to all types of combat, regardless of whether you grapple, strike or trap, throw or force your opponent down.

Principle #4 Principle #4 Economy of Movement

Two essential resources that you should save and make use of during combat or any other life-threatening situation such as energy and time. Efficiency of motion helps both. This principle of combat comes in Wing Chun as well as other combat art forms like fencing.

The goal is to employ the most straightforward and effective attacks and movements. It is not necessary to come up with any elaborate or fancy movements since in a street fight you won't have the time to practice a particular pose or wind-up. After you've finished performing your fancy, non-essential move your opponent could have grabbed the chair, stick, or something else and struck your with it.

If you apply this concept, you can gain clarity, simplicity and effectiveness. You'll think and behave in a straightforward manner. You will approach every scenario by determining the simplest and most efficient method to resolve any issue (or disperse a threat, for instance, if you're in a conflict).

Directness simply means that you perform things naturally. You don't have to bend or stretching in a non-natural way that leaves you un in a tizzy state or unprepared to take on or protect. It also means that you tackle every circumstance with discipline, always by using the most effective method.

Because you want to save energy and spend the shortest amount of time, your attacks should take the minimum amounts of effort. It is common to see JKD instructors and practitioners discuss making use of the "longest weapon to strike the nearest goal." Simply say, if your right fist is close to your opponent, you can use it to hit.

Keep in mind that you should be attacking the nearest possible target that is presented to you. Some attackers will start with a knee that is exposed which is why they will do an acrobatic side kick towards the knee. Others will strike you with a haymaker that will go as far as they will. This leaves their face open and close to your punch or your kick and then strike the face of the person who is in the lead (and naturally, it's also your most direct to hit). This is also true when your opponent attempts to strike and knock you down . He's in front of you with his face as you try to grab his legs, and then strike his face (use the knee, kick or even a jab).

Principiale #5 5 - Punch as well as Parry at the same time

The second principle comes of Wing Chun and it is utilized in various martial arts like Krav Maga (known as "bursting"). These martial arts require you to reduce your moves by parrying an attack and then countering the attack in the same moment.

Parrying isn't really an actual block. If you block a kick, punch or elbow strike, only one area of your body absorbs all the force of the attack. It is obvious that you'll still sustain any kind of injury when you resist an attack. If you block a punch, you'll only redirect or deflect it that the strike doesn't hit its target while the weapon (for example) simply passes through and moves across.

Your opponent is left open because he's to be focusing on reversing the attack he was launching. This is the perfect time to launch an attack. This method is obviously, but it is a long-term process that requires lots of practice.

Keep in mind this: Wing Chun was designed for women. They're usually less able to fight so they needed to come up with methods for women to defeat opponents with minimal force, and in the quickest possible speed. So, the combination of punch and parry is a good idea in real fights. there is always somebody stronger, more powerful and more powerful than you.

Bruce Lee himself wasn't a massive or tall person. He needed to come up with an approach to defeat larger and more powerful opponents. Parrying is a strategy because he didn't have the strength or the size to absorb each punch that was thrown at him. Additionally, he developed an excellent sense of timing, too.

Principle #6 - Stop Hits

If you think that simultaniously punching and parrying is an innovative concept for martial art, then you haven't yet seen anything. Stop-hits actually increase the intensity. Bruce Lee is known for staying away from his adversaries.

You can observe this from his fight and film videos. He once stated also:

"To get to me, you have to move towards me. Your attack gives me the opportunity to capture you."

Be aware of your strike range and you can see the opponent's plans to strike. Similar is true for all combat arts. For example, boxers tend to keep their opponents out of range. If they want their opponent to strike their opponent with punches,, they must make a move.

What you do and how you react is when the stop hit takes place. In the event that your time to react isn't fast the opponent has already taken the step to get close to you and then thrown the punch. The only option available to you at this point is to stop the punch . If you're quick enough, you could also counter and parry.

A better choice in an inning of striking is to take a stop hit. Be aware of the signals of your opponent. If you step forward with your right foot indicates that the punch is coming towards you. A hip turn could mean an attack. If your opponent is able to duck down, he could be looking to takedown.

These movements, which are pre-planned, provide opportunities for you to hit and keep your opponent off his feet. It's to be pure science (and somewhat easy and practical, too) but even JKD practitioners admit that it is among the abilities that are the most difficult to master. In movies, Bruce Lee can easily take out an opponent using an arcing house kick on the head, while the opponent was ready to leap into the air to kicks or another move.

Before you can learn stop hits you need to first integrate efficiency of movement as simultaneously punching and parrying (defense and offense in one movement). Keep in mind that the concept of stop hits isn't an original teaching method. It's been around for quite some time now and is a part of fencing and Wing Chun (i.e. their masters have been doing it from the beginning). Simply put, it's something that is attainable, but it takes a amount of time and practice to master this technique or principle.

Principle #7 - Combat Realism

One of the fundamentals of JKD is combat realistic. Each technique you master and every exercise you do as well as every training session is designed to be geared towards realistic fighting situations in real reality. It is possible to say that this can be described as one of many major reasons that JKD isn't really suited to compete in MMA.

In the world of fight sports rules safeguard and restrict fighters. That's where their weaknesses are. A person who has been familiar with fighting in sporting events may believe that the real world is also governed by rules. They are at a disadvantage as in the real world there aren't any rules.

The adrenaline is rushing in and you're being dragged around you are unable to remember any complicated martial art technique that you were taught at the training gym. You also have the illusion of tunnel vision. You only see the man who is in front of you. it's hard to see the guys to your side who want to hurt you. There is no fancy footwork or hand movements are required in that situation. At times like this the most basic method of defense or attack is used.

It's no longer a game or merely waiting to earn points. Every strike you take in combat real-time should be taken seriously - it must be fatally injured or even knock out your opponent. In circumstances of life or death take out the make sure to kill. You should be able to do this in a matter of seconds with the least quantity of work.

The basis of realistic combat is the concept that Bruce Lee taught as "aliveness." He stated famously "boards don't strike back." In training together, you and your instructor will utilize and put on the most effective forms of protective gear, so you can practice striking at full contact (or nearly full contact, according to the circumstances).

This will allow JKD students to train in real-world scenarios and learn how to strike and be hit in real-life situations while maintaining a high degree of security. Anything less than that is pretending to have the skills to defend yourself when you actually do not know how things actually are in a real-life fight with someone who truly wants to smudge you off your feet.

Principiale #8 Center Line Theory

The principle, as mentioned earlier straight in Wing Chun. What do you think is the central line? Imagine a line beginning at the top of the head, and then going through the stomach, chest, and groins of a person sitting right in the front of you. The space that the line passes through is the center of that person's body.

The center is the most important aspect to gaining advantage in position when you're in a battle. When it comes to Wing Chun, the idea is to control, dominate and take advantage of the opponent's center or middle line. A fighter who can control his center line and the center line of his opponents gain an advantage. Your opponent will be able to do little attacking or defense on the side. Because you are in the center (close distance combat) so all your strikes will hit first.

Three guidelines for controlling centerline:

1. You can control an opponent's line of center by taking over it.

2. Guard your center.

3. Make sure you take advantage of your opponent's center to keep the upper hand.

4. The fighter who has control of the centerline is in the lead and is in control of the fight.

Chapter 13: Jeet Kune Do Combat Ranges

The Four Fundamental Ranges

Now we're moving into less familiar water. Many people have heard about the four main ranges found in Jeet Kune Do. In the past the four different ranges that combat can be integrated into the modern mixed martial art. Bruce Lee taught that training within these four ranges can distinguish JKD from other types that are martial.

He also referred to other martial arts that focus mostly on two or three ranges. JKD participants are instructed and trained to combat in the four ranges, not only two. The basic ranges have evolved and evolved over time. They were previously known as medium range, long variety, short range and short range.

But, they are often unclear, so they must be identified with different names in order to be more specific. The new names for the categories are the punching range, kicking range range and grappling area.

Punching Range

The range of punches is the distance you have to travel to cover in order to hit your opponent's box with a punch. JKD students learn to use a variety of punches. Of course, the punches are different in accordance with the form of martial art. For example Karate punches are generally chambered (i.e. being derived from a chambered stance) and the same technique can be taught by other martial art, such as kung fu or Tae kwon Do. The straight punch boxing punch is a direct strike with the boxing arm on top of the rear of your foot. The strength behind the straight strike comes from the rotational motion of your hips that carry the weight of the whole body.

Some punches are faster than other punches. We'll look at the types of punches suggested by JKD in a subsequent chapter. Keep in mind the fact that Bruce Lee taught that when you have to punch, hit, however if you're required to kick or employ any other weapon , then you can utilize it. Use whatever is at your disposal.

Kicking Range

The range of kicking is more expansive in comparison to the punching range. A kick, as per an unofficial definition, requires making use of hip, foot and tibia, the heel and the thighs. In some cases, the knees can also be used in order to kick (it is often referred to as the knee strike).

Kicking has been used since the time of commemoration. It's difficult to track the development of this particular form of combat since a variety of martial arts across the globe utilize it. Certain kicks are employed to harm your opponent while some are employed to distract or displace.

We will discuss the most basic suggested kicks for JKD athletes in a separate chapter. Take note the fact that Bruce Lee is famous for his quick, precise kicks that eliminate opponents quickly. When your adversary is in kicking the distance, then you can kick.

Trapping Range

Trapping isn't to confuse with the grappling. Trapping is a form of clinch fighting technique that is effective in close quarter-fights. The trapping techniques employed in JKD originate origins in Wing Chun - remember that Bruce Lee was a student of the famous Wing Chun master Yip Man.

The two JKD along with Wing Chun practitioners make use of hand trapping and forearm techniques. The various techniques employed by both martial arts are tan-sao (hand blocking using the palm raised) and lap sao (hand gripping techniques) as well as the pak Sao (slap blocking) and many more.

The aim of trapping isn't to simply block , or even prepare your opponent for throwing. The main reason you should use trapping is to prepare the opponent to be able to launch a swift and quick counter sometimes with multiple counter-attacks. This is exactly the same way to go every time you're caught in a clinch with the Muay boxer or boxer. The aim is to position your opponent to strike the next time.

Grappling Range

It's interesting to note that most street fights end being on the floor. If you're at a bar or in any other place where you're involved in a fight, it's likely the fight will be on the ground with you sitting on top or the other person sitting standing on top of you, ready to smack you in the face.

Grappling simply is the use of different strategies and counter-maneuvers you can employ to control the opponent, subdue, and even sometimes fracture the joints of your opponent. It is possible to use grappling techniques to push a bigger and more powerful opponent to the ground , providing you with a superior position regardless of your physical handicap.

3 Different Variations

Apart from the immediate four ranges previously, JKD practitioners are also taught to combat in three additional areas: high, mid and low. The high range includes attacks that target the shoulders and all the way to the head. The mid-range includes attacks on the torso, and any other part in that zone. The lower range includes attacks from the waist upwards.

JKD students are taught to perform attacks that target the three. Of course, there is an idea and a basis for the use of these different options. The concept is to study your opponent's position on which range that he feels most comfortable in. If you observe that he is most likely to attack the head or the high end, then you are able to counter him on the two other ranges which are generally not covered.

On the other hand, there are instances where you do not have the opportunity to evaluate your opponent. Certain fights start suddenly and without warning. If this is the situation, then the best strategy is to utilize the distance that's exposed to engage. If your opponent grabs an empty wine bottle and raises his arm above his head , the face of your opponent is exposed. strike from the high-range.

If your opponent is destined with a punch, but leave his crotch open, then strike from the low distance. Certain opponents like to stand in a wide position and spread their feet wide and their calves and knees are exposed - then strike low. The opponent hides his face when he attempts to walk forward and slither towards you - perhaps to clinch, or a bear hug. Locate the area that's open and strike. It could be the stomach, which is open, or the foot is taking the next step and waiting for your to sweep your own foot , and then set up for a throw.

Chapter 14: Punches

It can be said you can say that Jeet Kune Do is primarily the stand-up kind of art. Much of the focus in this system of fighting centers around interception. In this article, we'll discuss some of the most basic hand techniques (mainly hand strikes and punches) that are taught by JKD practitioners. Many of them appear simple, but everybody should be able to recognize the practical and practical application of these techniques.

Keep in mind that as Bruce Lee developed these hand techniques, and the other techniques discussed in this book they were framed from the perspective of the weaker fighter that is at the disadvantage. This means that these techniques could be utilized and in the toughest fights.

JKD is kicking in the punch.

Bruce Lee taught that in jeet kune do there aren't any direct attacks. This means that your strikes, whether they are for defense or offense, will be countered or following an attack or feint. You'll be able to master a number of feints to prepare your opponent for the martial arts.

Combating principles such as deceit timing, strategy and speed are at the foundation to the technique of strike in JKD. An expert in this art of fighting blends all these concepts and provides opportunities to strike and beat the opponent.

You can't strike a blow and expect it to hit your opponent's forehead when your opponent's guard is raised. It is likely that your opponent will simply avoid or block your punch which will spend your time and energy. Also, you are leaving your opponent open to counterattacks in the event that you throw punches on the spur of the moment.

There has to be intention and a reason behind every punch you take. Correctly timed punches should be used and utilized based on the actions of your opponent and the opponent's inaction. For instance, if your opponent pulls away from you and leaves a clear line of attack towards his chin, it is an indication of a positive attack with an uppercut or straight kick at your opponent's face.

When your opponent's reaction is slow to every move you make will give you an indication regarding the appropriate speed and timing that you must employ to take advantage of his sluggish responses. The general rule is that your tactics must be influenced by the defense that your opponent is employing.

Compound Attacks

The attack in JKD is likely to come as an attack that is compound. When you think of it in terms of colloquial it is important not to have all your eggs into one basket. Don't invest all your energy into one strike, kick or knockdown attempts. The skilled fighter who is trying to beat a skilled opponent will attempt to deceive and outsmart his opponent.

A compound attack should always require a pre-action. It doesn't necessarily have to be a mix of punches or a mix of strikes. Keep in mind that in a real fighting on the streets, you do not have to rely on jabs to force your opponent to reveal his weaknesses. This is certainly true in the boxing ring, in which only punches are permitted. However, in the real world you can employ almost anything to confuse and make your opponent think. You can therefore use any hand strike that is most efficient. One example could be the hand jab.

Hand Technique #1 - Finger Jab

For mixed martial arts as well as other forms of fighting, looking into at the opponent's eyes is considered a sin. This is one of the reasons why they wear closed gloves as well as the standard MMA gloves are opened to let your fingers loose. It's more comfortable when you are looking to wrestle your opponent, however eye pokes are not legal actions in MMA.

Image Credit Bruce Lee's Fighting Method (Lee, Uyehara)

This is the reason there aren't a lot of JKD practitioners taking part in MMA. Mixed martial arts, as well as other types of competition fighting is not street combat. Sure, it can teach you to punch and box, grapple and fight, but the scenario which you're currently in won't provide any real-world fighting situations.

A poke in the eye can appear as a surprise. The first reaction to such attacks is to evade or avoid it. It will make us vulnerable for a subsequent attack. In JKD the leading finger jab is among the primary lines of attack or defense. The other primary offenses include knee kicks and an shin kick. we'll cover in the future.

As opposed to a closed-fisted strike, a finger provides you with an extra few inches to get closer to your opponent. It's not just an annoying attack that may make your opponent feel unbalanced however, it's quicker and can reach your opponent earlier.

"The on guard stance"

Finger jabs are thrown towards the on guard posture. If you're right handed, your leading arm will be the right arm, and your right foot will move towards the front. Your left hand and left leg and arm will fall behind. Your right hand is at ease and relaxed - ready to strike when needed. However, this hand may also be slightly extended in front of your opponent.

Making the Finger Jab

It is possible to throw the finger as you would throw the regular jabs in boxing. Simply move your arm forward very quickly. Also, you must take a one step forward using your leading foot (right foot if the right-handed). In contrast to a boxing jab your fingers will become extended as you hit this punch.

The main focus of this jab will be the eyes of your opponent. If you raise your arms in order to attack your opponent, make sure you keep an even line between your nose and your hands. This will ensure that you're not delivering a straight punch. By doing this you're throwing an unintentional strike from your center. This is extremely fast and hard to ignore or even detect at times.

No Direct Attacks

As I mentioned in the past, there aren't direct assaults in JKD. You can't use a finger jab as you do in boxing. Jabs are typically thrown by boxers as Hail Mary strikes hoping they'll hit on their opponents or force them to change direction to open up. This is not how the jab is executed or utilized in JKD.

You may either allow your opponent to start the preparation stage prior to striking, which allows you the opportunity to strike directly before your opponent has started his attack, or to try to make your opponent open up defenses.

As an example, you could lower your body to appear make an uppercut or strike the opponent's middle section. This will trigger him to drop his guard and leave his high-range (i.e. shoulders to heads) ready for an attack immediately.

This feint can be done by using either your left hand or right hand. Be aware that you shouldn't throw your finger leading strike without anticipating the reaction of your opponent. If your opponent drops his guard after you've ducked and strike forward, you should make a forward strike using the right side of your hand (left hand in the case of left-handed) and target the eyes. Naturally, during play, your opponent is wearing equipment for the head that provides an element of protection for eyes. There's no need to worry about causing injury to the eyes of your opponent.

Hand Technique #2 - Straight Lead

Straight lead punches have been mentioned in this book numerous times before. As mentioned earlier, it is similar to jabs, but you'll use the lead hand. If you're right-handed the right hand will do the majority task. For JKD practitioners leading straights are frequently described as "the bread-and-butter" of the martial art.

A lead straight punch is the most popular due to its speed and precise. It also only requires a brief distance to get to its intended target. Take note that, just like a jab the straight lead punch isn't going to take out anyone in a single hit. With the addition of weight, as any jab straight leads, they generate more power than the regular boxing jab.

The jab, like jabs has two main uses. It is the first. You can use it to determine the range of your punch. It is possible to determine the extent of you can punch by applying the lead straight. This is why you could also utilize this tool to maintain your adversaries in or within your range of punching. Another benefit of the straight lead punch is to prepare the next punch.

The Lead Straight

Image Credit Bruce Lee's Fighting Method (Lee, Uyehara)

Certain MMA fighters are also known to use the lead straight without realizing it. Here's an example Georges St. Pierre throwing an open straight at Josh Koscheck. It is not uncommon to hear announcers at the ringside call "stiff jab" or "stiff jab" but it's whatever it's called, regardless of what you name it.

Keep in mind that you must keep it simple and is clear. There are a variety of ways to throw an oblique lead. Some individuals prefer to rotate their hips, while others shift their weight. It is possible to use the dominant hand for throwing it and throw it using a non-dominant hand. Whatever method you choose to use for the "stiff jab" keep in mind what it's for and utilize it whenever necessary.

Chapter 15: Basic Jeet Kune Do Kicks

Your legs are obviously longer than your arms and are also more powerful. In the previous chapter of this book, it is stated that the finger jab is among the most important tools you can employ to defend against or take on your adversary. In this chapter, we'll take a explore the jabs that are given by JKD students and the way they can be utilized as the primary tool to defend and attack an adversary (or an entire group of adversaries).

Kicks in JKD

The best kicks to use in jeet kune do are ones that are quick and require minimal movement. The more straight an attack is, the better it'll be. This means that kicks that spin around, and appear to be dancing are not recommended.

In JKD the best kick to deliver is one you can throw before your opponent has the chance to defend. A kick that hits before your opponent reacts is the best. Keep in mind to kick, you will be committing yourself to it, and this basically takes you unbalanced because you'll only be with one foot.

Make sure you are committed to your kick - this means that you must throw the ball in a way that has a significant amount of anxiety and enthusiasm behind it. Keep in mind that some opponents might attempt to grab your kicking leg. To stop them from doing this it is important to frighten your opponent by using your movements or other strikes prior to delivering swift, sharp strong kick.

There are three crucial moments when you throw a kick that you must pay attention to when throwing your kick, landing, and recovery. In JKD kicks, those that move forward with the motion of knees are suggested. Certain of these kicks can be somewhat similar to chambered-type kicks from taekwondo or karate (though they are not chambered) but not the sweeping kicks that are used for Muay Thai athletes.

There are no chambering actions in JKD. The transition from one phase to the next is one fluid movement.

As an JKD practitioner, you'll be taught to kick and then shift either forward or backwards, moving laterally, or even circle with your adversaries. Let's begin with one the longest-lasting weapons that is the most effective knee kicks as well as the leading shin kicks.

Shin Kick and Knee Kick

A side kick to the shin or the knee is among the primary kicks utilized in JKD particularly when you're battling an opponent for the very first time. These are extremely hazardous kicks, and can be extremely destructive as you could snap your opponent's knees if the kick is executed correctly.

Everyone seems to be getting the notion that if you are kicked in the knees or shins and then kicks your shin, they're trying to kill you. This deters your opponents from moving forward, and you are able to limit the distance even if you've never hit this punch a number of times. This will allow you to assess the distance and determine the way of fighting your opponent. This is particularly useful in fights on the street in which your opponents don't meet you until they are introduced to the other.

How to Throw a Sidekick at either the Shin or Knee

To throw a sidekick correctly to the knee or shin you must shift your body in the direction of your opponent before you launch the strike. It's important to remember that you shouldn't simply turn and kick, your opponent is able to detect the movements of your opponent and then counter return to the submission to hold, or even throw.

It is possible to begin your move by making a slight feint , or move in such as to make your opponent think. You can, for instance, strike a right-handed strike (assuming that you're right-handed) or a right-finger jab if you locate an opening to that punch. The goal is to distract your opponent. Turn to the left, then extend your right leg while keeping your right foot in a vertical position (i.e. in a straight line to the ground with your toes pointed towards the side).

The goal of this kick is the shin or knee whichever is the nearest to the target. Here's an example this kick performed by Anderson Silva, one of the UFC's most feared fighters:

In MMA the kick can be described as linear knee strike or simply a push at the knee. The knee of the opponent gets stretched and, if you perform the kick correctly it will deliver sufficient force that breaks the knee of your opponent.

Bruce Lee sometimes tricks his opponents into believing he's about strike high when raising his arms like Bruce Lee is about to jump into the air, and then kick high. In their shock the opponents are hit with swift and powerful punches to the knee or shin, which causes them to lose balance. The fight is ended.

The leading side kick

A side kick can be thought of as the strongest strike that anyone could deliver in JKD. The side kick is so potent it even when your adversary is able to stop it you can be sure that he'll suffer significant harm. A few of the players who attempted to stop the kick ended up falling across the floor or simply fall to the floor, writhing in pain.

The force and amount of discomfort that you will experience from the kick will be determined by the area of your body that your foot is placed on. Side kicks already produce lots of power when it is thrown from a medium distance. It could produce more power when throwing it from a greater distance.

It is possible to throw a lead side kick to different parts of your body. For example, you could throw a leading side kick to a player who attacks the ball from some distance, aiming at your rib cage.

Hook Kick

Hook kicks are a middle distance kick that is regarded as a dominant kick because it can be utilized to hit a target quite quickly. The hook kick is extremely versatile because it can be utilized to strike the groin or midsection and even the head. In other styles of martial arts it is known as the round kick. It is known as "hook kick" within JKD due to the fact that the path that the foot follows is exactly the similar to the line you follow by your fist during throwing the hook or cross.

This is how you can throw the hook kick. Start in the on guard posture with your right hand leading, and the left foot being the one to follow (assuming that you're right-handed). You move your foot that is trailing you forward, and then raise your leading leg while keeping the knee bent as if you are chambering. You then use your kicking leg to kick your foot towards your goal (extending the leg). The angle or height that you kick will differ based on the goal you are trying to reach.

After you extend your leg, you must quickly retract it and place your foot back onto the earth. Then, you must return to the starting point or in a guarded position. Make sure to complete all that in one smooth motion, to ensure that you don't lose yourself in the course of your move.

Tips: Make sure to move on your left side and your hips as you deliver the kick. The more force you apply to your kick, and the faster you kick, the kick, the more force you can generate to your kick.

Bruce Lee performing a high hook kick

Bruce Lee demonstrating a hook kick to the head

Stop Kick

Stop kicks in JKD is like side kicks towards the shin or side kick for the knee. The major different is that the kick in JKD is delivered more high. It can be used at the medium range, as well as the distance. It's no surprise that this kick is powerful enough to deter a raging enemy. It's not just about kicking the opponent; you're actually striking him down with this kick. This kick is an actual thrust which directly hits the opponent. It is also used in situations where you need to avoid attacks and perform some side-slipping.

Bruce Lee demonstrating a stop kick

Image credit Bruce Lee's Fighting Method (Lee, Uyehara)

Chapter 16: Different Kinds Of Tae Kwon Do

Similar to the other forms, there are varieties of Tae Kwon Do. Different schools offer different methods and methods, or even the identical ones, but with different variants that are their own. There are three main kinds of TKD that are:

- Word Taekwondo Federation (WTF)

International Taekwon-Do Federation (ITF)

- Tang Soo Do Forms

Word Taekwondo Federation (WTF) Patterns

They WTF Tae Kwon Do sequences are quick, simple and speedy. They aren't easy to master, particularly the first one however, with practice one can ease into the routine. They have 8 sequences in them that are similar to other ones however they have different methods, and it is crucial not to mix them up with one the other. They include:

- Taegeuk 1 - Taegeuk-il-jang

- Taegeuk 2 - Taegeuk-e-jang

- Taegeuk 3 - Taegeuk-sam-jang

- Taegeuk 4 - Taegeuk-sah-jang

- Taegeuk 5 - Taegeuk-oh-jang

- Taegeuk 6 - Taegeuk-yuk-jang

- Taegeuk 7 - Taegeuk-chil-jang

- Taegeuk 8 - Taegeuk-pal-jang

It is crucial for students to be able to master all these types of forms. If they can master these kinds of sequences, they will be elevated to the highest degree. In order, each sequence is more complex and challenging than the previous one. If a student is able to master the eight sequences in a row and is able to pass the test, they are eligible as black belt.

International Taekwon-Do Federation (ITF) Patterns

The styles of the International Taekwon-Do Federation are more traditional. These patterns last longer, and demand more force. In ITF we have 24 patterns. These patterns are also known as "taekwondo hyung" or "tul. The initial patterns are exactly the same, except for different parts of our bodies. As they progress, they become more complicated and challenging. They are:

-- Chon Ji (Yellow Stripe Pattern)

-- Dan Gun (Yellow Belt Pattern)

- Do San (Green Stripe Pattern)

- Won Hyo (Green Belt Pattern)

" Yul Gok (Blue Stripe Pattern)

- Joong Gun (Blue Belt Pattern)

toi-gye (Red Stripe pattern)

- Hwa Rang (Red Belt Pattern)

-- Choong Moo (Black Stripe Pattern)

Because the moves may be similar and complex It is recommended not to be rushed. Do them slowly to ensure that you don't get confused by one move with another. It's not as important as perfect timing.

Tang Soo Do Forms

Tang Soo Do forms, often referred to Moo Do Kwan Taekwondo, are among the most exciting sequences. They affect our external and internal wellbeing. They assist us in achieving the qi energy in us as well as draw it out the maximum benefit the energy externally. Tang

Soo Do contain some traditional patterns, however Grandmaster Hwang Kee introduced several new forms too. The designs that make up Tang Soo Do include:

- Pyun Ahn Cho Dan

- Pyun Ahn E Dan

- Pyun Ahn Sam Dan

- Pyun Ahn Sah Dan

- Pyun Ahn Oh Dan

Bassi Bassi

-- Nai Han Ji Cho Dan

-- Nai Han Ji Ee Dan

- Nai Han Ji Sam Dan

Jin Do Do Jin Do

Lo Hai Hai Lo Hai

-

There are other patterns available, however if you are enrolled in an school or academy, none of them will be covered in your course.

Chapter 17: Tae Kwon Do Equipment

Although Tae Kwon Do is a martial art that is a non-armed type of combat, there's an array of tools that can be utilized to help you train and to learn faster. In schools and institutes, the proper equipment and equipment are essential to guarantee safety. It is imperative to purchase the best equipment that is not with inferior quality, since they last a long time, and fulfill their objective. There is a assumption among many that it is best to purchase cheaper equipment until you have learned the art of making it work; however, this is not the case. Equipment and gear are as essential for beginners and experts as professionals. Here is a list of Tae Kwon Do equipment and equipment:

Uniforms:

It is mandatory to wear uniforms for training. They permit free movement in combat and practice. You must wear at minimum three uniforms at any time so that if one is dirty, they can have another easily available.

Taekwondo Shoes

Taekwondo shoes differ from normal shoes in that they're completely lacing-free and perfectly fitting. They're also made in a way that they do not hinder the training or performance by adhering to the mat. A properly fitted shoe helps keep your legs in sync, which makes it appear more natural.

Practice Mats

The mats have many functions. First, they mark your boundaries, which are essential in Taekwondo tournaments. Additionally, they decrease the chance of injury in the event that you slip or fall during training.

Punching Bags

Punching bags are designed for those who would like to work at home. They help you improve your strike. Be sure to have a an adequate ceiling that will support the bag and support its weight prior to you purchase one.

Kicking Bags

For a better understanding of your kicks, buy bags to kick with. They are readily available at Tae Kwon Do teaching institutes and also at the Tae Kwon Do training institutes, however advanced players have one at home for work on their skills.

Re-breakable Boards

When doing Tae Kwon Do exercises, the participants are usually asked to break the boards through the power of their hand. Breakable boards that are only for one time like their namesake are designed for one time use only. A large number of them is costly, therefore you should consider buying breakable ones which can be broken then put back together again to be used again and again.

Other Equipment

There's plenty of equipment that can be useful in the field of Tae Kwon Do. You should have one that you own, since Taekwondo is exhausting and cause excessive sweating and causes you to drink water regularly. In addition, the Taekwondo shoes are very delicate and could become damaged or loose, therefore glue for your shoes can be useful. Apart from that it is possible to purchase Taekwondo-related books. It's more than just the art of fighting, but a way of life and the more you understand about it, the more you'll be able to comprehend it.

Chapter 18: Tae Kwon Do Kicks And Strikes

When you learn Tae Kwon Do, your instructor will instruct you on different strikes and kicks. Each strike and kick are accompanied by names that help you remember them since the movement and portion of your foot which strikes is different when striking, and is usually the area of the body that takes the strike. For example, when you kick on the rear, toes, and the foot's ball make the primary strike. Here is a list of the strikes and kicks:

Kicks

Naeryeo Chagi, or Axe Kick Naeryeo Chagi, also known as Axe Kick is used to strike the person on the head or the neck bone.

Dwi Chagi also known as the Back Kick This is a strong kick that is it is difficult to learn. It requires turning your body around 180 degrees while maintaining the leg in a straight line. For those who are new to the sport there are a few alternatives for this kick.

Ap Chai (also known as front Kick Front Kick is a fundamental kick that lets you punch your opponent beneath the face or into the groin.

Meereo Chagi or Push Kick The push kick can be effective when you're in the defensive. If it is properly landed and the opponent is knocked off balance.

Yeop Chagi, or the Side Kick Side Kick: another option to use to defend yourself. It is most effective when you target the knee of your opponent.

Although these are just one or two kicks, there are many more to learn on the way, such as Kicks like the Butterfly Kick, Shin Kick, Scissor Kick, Flying Kick, Crescent Kick, Roundhouse Kick, as well as a variety of variations on these kicks.

Strikes

Tae Kwon Do is not solely about punches. It also requires a lot of hand skill and there are a variety of punches and strikes that have to be learned during the process of training. These include:

Jab: A quick and easy punch, and one of the first to be taught in the basics class, assists you keep your opponent from getting away.

Upper Cut: During an event or fight in a fight, an upper cut can cause a serious injury on the lower jaw and ribs.

Hammer Fist: it is a powerful punch that is surprisingly simple. The fist is locked but instead of striking on the knuckles' side it is struck using the padded side (the part of your pinky) like you would do when you turn your hand into the shape of a Hammer.

Elbow Strike: An elbow strike is, without doubt, among the most powerful strikes to strike when fighting with your hands. The bones that line the elbows are much larger than the bones of your fist, allowing you to deliver extremely powerful strikes.

There are a variety of different strikes could be learned, like Palm Heel Strike, Tiger Claw, Knife Hand Strike, Ridge Hand Strike, Spear Hand, Rear Arm Punch as well as others. It is essential to get plenty of practice prior to performing these techniques in combat, or else you risk serious injury to your hands or bones that could prevent you from doing it again.

Chapter 19: The Trainings For Tae Kwon Do

Tae Kwon Do requires a healthy mind and a sturdy body. It is important to work your body to improve its strength and flexibility for better performance during Tae Kwon Do contests. To accomplish this you can do a variety of exercises that you could do that target a specific portion of your body so that your body is strengthened. The exercises you could do include:

Chest Dips:

This is an exercise you must do in order to strengthen your chest. Apart from strengthening the chest strength, it will also help to strengthen your upper body. A dip station as well as a the weight belt are essential for this workout.

Bench Press:

This exercise is designed to work the chest and also the triceps muscle of the arms and shoulder deltoid muscles. For this workout.

Triceps Kickbacks:

It is a great exercise for triceps that involves approximately 90% the muscle's activity. When you do this exercise, you'll work against gravity, which is why it can be quite difficult. If weights are limiting your movement, feel at ease using lighter ones. It doesn't matter how heavy the weights that you workout with however the level of performance you are able to do the movements.

Pull-Ups:

Pull-Ups are an excellent exercise to build your muscles and punches. It's simple to do and anyone can do it. The only thing you need is a pull-up bar which must be put in place or repaired at the time of installation.

Push-Ups:

They are crucial because they help strengthen the upper body. There are a variety of variations of push-ups which maximize their benefits, but they can be tiring also. Push-ups with elevated incline, Diamond push-ups, Plyometric push-ups are the most well-known varieties, but it's recommended to begin by doing the basic push-ups. When you are able to perform the standard push-ups correctly, then you can begin to experiment and switch between the various variations of push-ups.

Woodchops:

It is an excellent exercise if you are looking to strengthen abdominal muscles and your back simultaneously. It helps improve flexibility of the spine and makes it stronger, which is beneficial since it allows you to execute many strikes and kicks quickly and efficiently. It's a vigorous exercise and is used by people who participate in squash, golf or other sports. because it helps restore balance to the body.

Bird Dog:

The exercise is designed to strengthen the butt and thighs, abdominal muscles and lower back. It can initially be difficult to maintain your balance when doing this exercise. However, when you master the control of your balance, the exercise is easy.

There are other exercises you could do as well. The aim is to strengthen all of the major areas of the body which participate in combat or affect fighting or affect fighting in some way. Don't do too much during any exercise. Practice slowly at a slower pace, and then, gradually, you can try the more advanced versions of exercises listed in the previous paragraphs.

Russian Twists, Vertical Leg Crunch along with Segmental Rotation workouts are suggested.

Chapter 20: Belts Of Tae Kwon Do

The belts of Tae Kwon Do serve as an indicator of ranking. In addition to ranks they also represent an important thing. Belts are an grading system, and they also have stripes. To go from a white belt to a yellow belt, you must first acquire the yellow stripe. Let's examine what belts from Tae Kwon Do mean and symbolise, and the their rank is.

White Belt

A while belt represents innocence. It's the start of the stage and every player starts with this belt automatically. It also serves as a motivating goal, by letting students know that the very best of them began with that white belt.

Before obtaining the yellow belt, one must have an orange stripe that goes through the grades.

Yellow Belt

The yellow belt represents earth. As students gain knowledge the earth symbolises an indication of them being an organism that continues to grow and increase. This belt follows called the green belt and requires two grades after receiving an orange belt to move to green belt. The grades are presented by way lines on the belt.

Green Belt

The green belt is a symbol of plants. In this case, the plant represents your taekwondo ability that is starting to grow and develop. Certain places are equipped with an orange belt in place of green. Another belt to consider is the blue one to be able to attain it, and one must pass two levels. One grade forms a blue line along the belt. The subsequent grade is the blue belt.

Blue Belt

A blue belt represents the sky. The sky is limitless according to them. The belt is a way to encourage you by letting the plant know how it's growing, and is required to continue to grow until it can reach the skies above. Next is called the red belt. Similar to other belts, two grades are required. The first result in stripes on the current belt while the second leads to the red belt.

Red Belt

Red belt symbolizes danger. This belt speaks towards the reality that the child is becoming extremely proficient at their craft however, it can be dangerous as well. At this stage the student is two years away from earning the black belt.

Black Belt

Black belts symbolize wisdom and bravery. It is a symbol of self-control for the student as well as their courage when faced with darkness and strength. It's not just about skill, but understanding the ways of life and also the way of life. The students are experts in their abilities, body and the mind. They exhibit control and discipline, but are prepared to fight when the need arises. The black belt also informs students and other participants that their journey to self-improvement is over.

When one has achieved the Black Belt, one has to keep practicing. It's not necessarily the final stage of the process but the beginning of an entirely new and improved way of living.

Chapter 21: Tae Kwon Do Basics

To learn an art, you have to understand the fundamentals. When one has a complete grasp of the fundamentals that one is able to comprehend the complexity that are involved in the practice. Tae Kwon Do basics are intended to assist those who are beginning to study this art to grasp a fundamental understanding of the art. This chapter we'll look at different Tae Kwon Do stances.

Apkubi Seogi

Apkubi Seogi can be described as the fundamental front stance of Tae Kwon Do. It is often referred to as the 'long forward stance. Before you can begin fighting your opponent, you must to establish a solid foundation that can be found by this position. A solid base will allow you to defend yourself and also attack more effectively. With this stance it is best to place one leg forward, keeping the knee aligned with your toes. Your other foot is set toward the back, firm as well as straight and firm. The shoulders remain straight in a straight line, with the abs firmly with the spine straight when in this position. Be sure to keep your eyes in the direction of your eyes straight at your opponent.

Dwitkubi Seogi

Dwitkubi Seogi is another common posture, also known as the "back posture. In this type of position, one foot is placed in front and the other placed behind, facing the sideways direction, and in a straight line with your front leg. The feet are placed so they are on the same line which means that if you move your front foot completely back, it will touch the heels that is on the foot behind. The back foot shouldn't rotate at more than 90 degrees. The legs are bent during this stance with the burden placed in the rear foot giving more attacking power for those on the front. Be sure to keep your abs strong with your back straight and focus on the towards the future.

Juchun Seogi

Horse Riding Stance is another term used for Juchun Seogi because it resembles the posture. The legs are to the sides, similar to riding a horse. the feet are pointing forward when in this posture. The knees must be perfectly aligned together with your toes. The back stays straight, and the abs and other muscles are kept tight. This position can be challenging initially, but it becomes easier as time passes.

Conclusion

I hope this book has taught you the fundamentals of Taekwondo. I hope it has taught you some basic self-defense strategies so that you are safe and secure when you're traveling alone or are left behind.

If you live or are exposed to a potentially dangerous situation, I suggest you to learn more advanced Taekwondo techniques in order to remain secure.

Also, I would like you to remember that martial arts are not meant to give you an excuse to start or stay in fighting. They are meant to keep you safe from troubles. Be aware of the rules of Taekwondo. They will help and protect you in Taekwondo.

Thank you again for choosing this book . be in peace.

www.ingramcontent.com/pod-product-compliance
Lightning Source LLC
Chambersburg PA
CBHW071839080526
44589CB00012B/1052